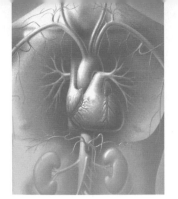

37.35

W9-BNP-765

BRYANLGH COLLEGE OF
HEALTH SCIENCES
Library Services

Invasive Hemodynamics in the Catheterization Laboratory: Self-Assessment and Review

Published by Remedica Publishing Limited
32–38 Osnaburgh Street, London, NW1 3ND, UK

Tel: +44 20 7388 7677
Fax: +44 20 7388 7457
Email: books@remedica.com
www.remedica.com

Publisher: Andrew Ward
In-house editor: Tamsin White
Design: Regraphica, London, UK

ISBN 1 901346 33 1
British Library Cataloguing-in Publication Data
A catalogue record for this book is available from the British Library

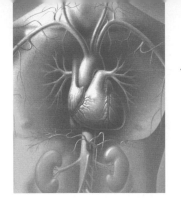

Invasive Hemodynamics
in the Catheterization Laboratory:
Self-Assessment and Review

Editors: Michael D Eisenhauer & Morton J Kern

REMEDICA
publishing

Contributors

Editors

Michael D Eisenhauer, MD, FACC, FACP
Chief, Cardiology Service, Department of Medicine
William Beaumont Army Medical Center
El Paso, Texas
Assistant Professor of Medicine,
Uniformed Services University of the Health Sciences
Bethesda, Maryland, USA

Morton J Kern, MD, FACC, FSCAI
Professor of Medicine, Cardiology Division, Department of Medicine
Director, J Gerard Mudd Cardiac Catheterization Laboratory
St. Louis University Health Sciences Center
St. Louis, Missouri, USA

Authors

Ellie Azrak, MD
Fellow in Cardiovascular Diseases
St. Louis University Health Sciences Center
St. Louis, Missouri, USA

Terry D Bauch, MD
Director, Cardiac Catheterization Laboratory
Brooke Army Medical Center
San Antonio, Texas, USA

Vincent S DeGeare, MD
Co-Director, Interventional Cardiology
Brooke Army Medical Center
San Antonio, Texas, USA

William C Dixon IV, MD
Fellow in Cardiovascular Diseases
Brooke Army Medical Center
San Antonio, Texas, USA

Amr El-Shafei, MD
Fellow in Cardiovascular Diseases
St. Louis University Health Sciences Center
St. Louis, Missouri, USA

James L Furgerson, MD
Staff Cardiologist
Brooke Army Medical Center
San Antonio, Texas, USA

Souheil Khouhaz, MD
Fellow in Cardiovascular Diseases
St. Louis University Health Sciences Center
St. Louis, Missouri, USA

Michael D Kwan, MD
Director, Congestive Heart Failure Service
Assistant Director, Cardiac Transplantation
Brooke Army Medical Center
San Antonio, Texas, USA

Kenneth LeClerc, MD
Director, Cardiac Rehabilitation
Brooke Army Medical Center
San Antonio, Texas, USA

Randolph Modlin, MD
Assistant Chief, Cardiology Service
Brooke Army Medical Center
San Antonio, Texas, USA

Martha Moore, MD
Fellow in Cardiovascular Diseases
St. Louis University Health Sciences Center
St. Louis, Missouri, USA

Carey L O'Bryan IV, MD
Fellow in Cardiovascular Diseases
Wilford Hall US Air Force Medical Center
San Antonio, Texas, USA

Mark Peele, MD
Director, Electrophysiology Service
Brooke Army Medical Center
San Antonio, Texas, USA

Karl C Stajduhar, MD
Chief, Cardiology Service
Brooke Army Medical Center
San Antonio, Texas, USA

Steven J Welka, DO
Fellow in Cardiovascular Diseases
Brooke Army Medical Center
San Antonio, Texas, USA

Joshua Winslow, MD
Fellow in Cardiovascular Diseases
Brooke Army Medical Center
San Antonio, Texas, USA

Preface

Much of our understanding of abnormalities of cardiac function is related to the genesis of pressure waveforms and blood flow. Hemodynamics remain fundamental to appreciating the clinical presentation of many cardiovascular disorders. Patients with acute myocardial infarction, valvular heart disease, constrictive physiology and left ventricular dysfunction are just a few syndromes that have distinct hemodynamic characteristics. In clinical practice, the examination of the pressure waveforms can assist in establishing diagnoses and treatment.

This book is a self-assessment and review of invasive hemodynamics. We have assembled a wide variety of common pressure waveforms and organized the material in a case review format with pertinent questions. The answers discuss interpretation of data, focusing on clinical findings that are helpful for clinical decision-making. This review is designed to stimulate thought and prepare the reader for questions that may be encountered on various board examinations. It is our hope that the questions and answers contain relevant didactic, as well as clinical, information and will provide the motivation for further study of hemodynamic problems in clinical practice.

This work was initiated by our continuing interest in hemodynamics in the catheterization laboratory. We recommend interested individuals review related materials in journals and publications, including Catheterization and Cardiovascular Interventions, Hemodynamic Rounds, 2nd edition, The Cardiac Catheterization Handbook and others appearing in the Suggested Reading section.

We gratefully acknowledge and appreciate the work of the contributors who provided focus on hemodynamic problems and formulated many of the questions to enhance the appreciation of these hemodynamic dilemmas. The editors thank Mrs Donna Sander and Ms Valerie Behrens for their diligent preparation of this text and express thanks to the cardiology staff and fellows-in-training at St. Louis University and Brooke Army Medical Center in San Antonio, Texas, for their assistance.

Morton J Kern & Michael D Eisenhauer

A special note to our readers:

Despite our efforts to thoroughly proof-read and verify the accuracy of each of the questions, answers and comments made in this text, unfortunately errors can sometimes occur in the publication process. We regret any inconvenience that may result from perceived inaccuracies in the final published version.

The editors kindly request your assistance in notifying the publisher of any errors, such that they can be corrected in any future revisions or editions of this text.

In addition, we invite you to submit any interesting hemodynamic tracings or clinical correlative findings that might be included in the next edition of this text. If your suggestion is added to the next edition, you will receive a free press-release copy as an expression of our appreciation.

Thank you!

Michael D Eisenhauer, MD
Morton J Kern, MD

To: Remedica Publishing, 32–38 Osnaburgh Street, London NW1 3ND, UK.

From: ⎯⎯⎯⎯⎯⎯⎯⎯⎯⎯⎯⎯⎯⎯⎯⎯⎯⎯⎯⎯⎯⎯⎯⎯⎯⎯

⎯⎯⎯⎯⎯⎯⎯⎯⎯⎯⎯⎯⎯⎯⎯⎯⎯⎯⎯⎯⎯⎯⎯⎯⎯⎯⎯⎯⎯⎯⎯

⎯⎯⎯⎯⎯⎯⎯⎯⎯⎯⎯⎯⎯⎯⎯⎯⎯⎯⎯⎯⎯⎯⎯⎯⎯⎯⎯⎯⎯⎯⎯

Error(s) identified:

(1) Question #: ⎯⎯⎯⎯⎯⎯⎯⎯⎯⎯⎯⎯⎯⎯⎯⎯⎯⎯⎯⎯⎯

⎯⎯⎯⎯⎯⎯⎯⎯⎯⎯⎯⎯⎯⎯⎯⎯⎯⎯⎯⎯⎯⎯⎯⎯⎯⎯⎯⎯⎯⎯⎯

⎯⎯⎯⎯⎯⎯⎯⎯⎯⎯⎯⎯⎯⎯⎯⎯⎯⎯⎯⎯⎯⎯⎯⎯⎯⎯⎯⎯⎯⎯⎯

(2) Question #: ⎯⎯⎯⎯⎯⎯⎯⎯⎯⎯⎯⎯⎯⎯⎯⎯⎯⎯⎯⎯⎯

⎯⎯⎯⎯⎯⎯⎯⎯⎯⎯⎯⎯⎯⎯⎯⎯⎯⎯⎯⎯⎯⎯⎯⎯⎯⎯⎯⎯⎯⎯⎯

⎯⎯⎯⎯⎯⎯⎯⎯⎯⎯⎯⎯⎯⎯⎯⎯⎯⎯⎯⎯⎯⎯⎯⎯⎯⎯⎯⎯⎯⎯⎯

Suggested Reading

Baim DS, Grossman W. Cardiac Catheterization, Angiography, and Intervention.
6th ed. Baltimore: Williams & Wilkins, 2000.

Bonow RO, Carabello B, De Leon AC et al. ACC/AHA Guidelines for the Management of
Patients with Valvular Heart Disease. A Report of the American College of Cardiology/American
Heart Association Task Force on Practice Guidelines
(Committee on Management of Patients with Valvular Heart Disease). J Am Coll Cardiol
1998;32(5):486–588.

Braunwald E. Valvular Heart Disease. In: Braunwald E, editor. Heart Disease:
a Textbook of Cardiovascular Medicine. 5th ed. Philadelphia: WB Saunders Co., 1997:1054–8.

Kern MJ, Deligonul U, Gudipati C. Hemodynamic and ECG Data. In: The Cardiac
Catheterization Handbook, 3rd ed. St. Louis: Mosby-Year Book, Inc., 1999:123–223.

Kern MJ. Hemodynamic Rounds. 2nd ed. New York: John Wiley & Sons, Inc., 1999.

Pepine CJ, Hill JA, Lambert CR. Diagnostic and Therapeutic Cardiac Catheterization. 3rd ed.
Baltimore: Williams and Wilkins, 1997.

Uretsky Barry F. Cardiac Catheterization: Concepts, Techniques and Applications. Malden
Massachusetts: Blackwell Science, 1997.

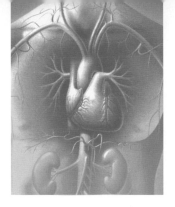

Contents

To Margaret and Anna Rose.
MJK

For my son, Sean, who has taught me there are so many more important things in life.
MDE

Chapter 1
Normal Hemodynamics

During normal respiration, the following right atrial (RA) pressures (Figures 1.1 and 1.2) were recorded.

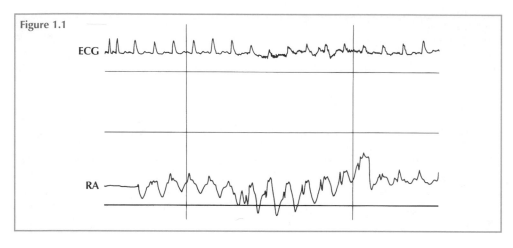

Figure 1.1

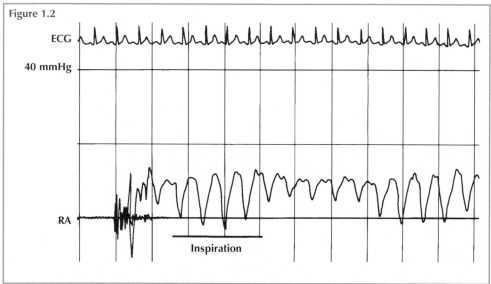

Figure 1.2

1. **Which tracing demonstrates a normal response?**
   a. Figure 1.1
   b. Figure 1.2

2. **What is the name of the phenomenon exhibited in Figure 1.2?**
   a. Duroziez's sign
   b. Müller's maneuver
   c. Kussmaul's sign
   d. Pulsus paradoxus
   e. Cannon A-wave

3. RA pressure is measured in a 68-year-old man with increasing shortness of breath at rest and on exertion (Figure 1.3). This pressure waveform is consistent with which of the following diagnoses?

    a. Myocardial ischemia
    b. Pericarditis
    c. Pulmonary hypertension
    d. Tricuspid regurgitation
    e. Congestive heart failure or constrictive physiology

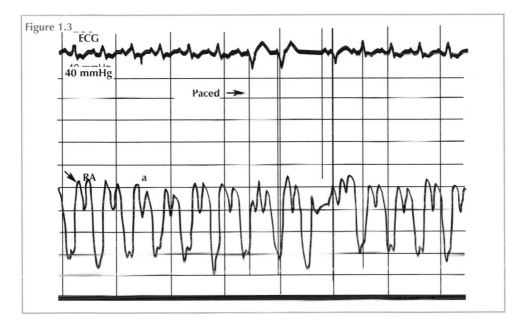

Figure 1.3

4. In a patient with a structurally normal heart, the RA pressure is always lower than the left atrial (LA) pressure.

    a. True
    b. False

5. Match the RA waveform tracings labeled 1–4 in Figure 1.4 with the clinical condition below:
    a. Constrictive pericarditis
    b. Tricuspid stenosis
    c. Normal
    d. Tricuspid regurgitation

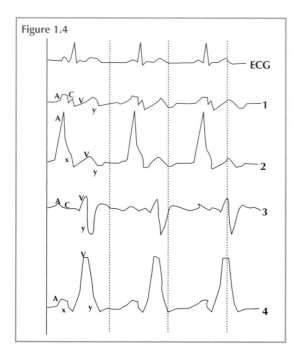

Figure 1.4

Simultaneous hemodynamic tracings of femoral artery (FA) pressure—taken through the side arm of the 8F sheath—and central aortic (Ao) pressure are shown. Central Ao pressure is obtained through the 7F pigtail catheter near the Ao valve (Figure 1.5). The tracings in the lower panel are obtained after crossing the Ao valve with the pigtail catheter.

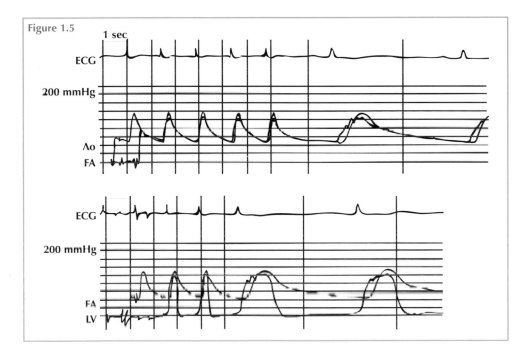

Figure 1.5

6. With regard to the hemodynamics in Figure 1.5, FA pressure is always higher than Ao pressure.
    a. True
    b. False

7. FA pressure is higher than Ao pressure because of:
    a. Increased systemic compliance
    b. Pressure transmission delay time
    c. Pressure waveform summation
    d. Hardening of the aorta and peripheral arteries
    e. Decreased systemic compliance

8. In Figure 1.6, the V-wave of the pulmonary capillary wedge (PCW) pressure is usually delayed relative to the left ventricular (LV) down stroke by:
   a. 10–20 msec
   b. 20–30 msec
   c. 40–120 msec
   d. 200–400 msec
   e. >500 msec

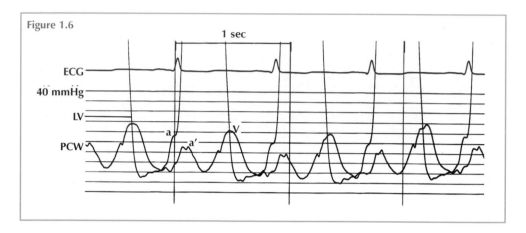

Figure 1.6

A 49-year-old man undergoing cardiac catheterization for a heart murmur and dyspnea on exertion has FA and LV pressures measured during a provocative maneuver.

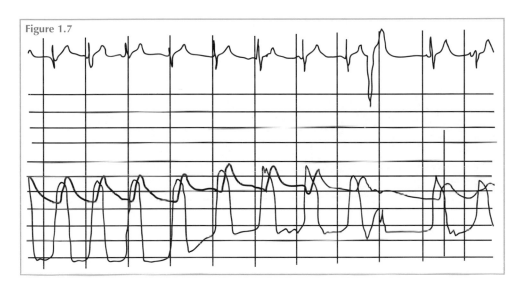

Figure 1.7

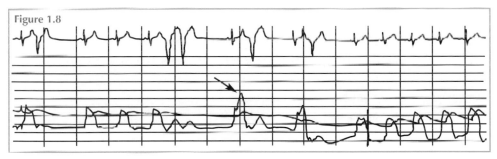

Figure 1.8

9. The maneuver on the hemodynamic tracings in Figures 1.7 and 1.8 is:
   a. Handgrip
   b. Valsalva's
   c. Müller's
   d. Squatting
   e. Amyl nitrate inhalation

10. In Figure 1.8, a patient with hypertrophic cardiomyopathy (HCM) develops ectopy during Valsalva's maneuver. What is the explanation for the increased LV–Ao gradient post-premature ventricular contraction (PVC)? See arrow.
    a. Increased systemic afterload (decreased LV compliance)
    b. Increased LV filling volume and pressures
    c. Decreased venous return (decreased preload)
    d. Volume shunting between right and left ventricle
    e. This patient does not have HCM, but does have fixed Ao stenosis

11. Which of the following best describes the hemodynamic response to aerobic exercise?

	CO	SVR	MAP
a.	↑	↓	↓
b.	↑	↓	↑
c.	↑	↓	↑↑
d.	↑	↑	↑↑
e.	↓	↑	↑

CO: cardiac output; MAP: mean arterial pressure;
SVR: systemic vascular resistance.

12. The increase in cardiac output, which accompanies exercise in the unconditioned subject, is best explained by which of the following:
a. A large increase in stroke volume and a large increase in heart rate
b. A modest increase in stroke volume and a large increase in heart rate
c. A large increase in stroke volume and a modest increase in heart rate
d. A modest decrease in stroke volume and a large increase in heart rate
e. A modest decrease in stroke volume and a modest increase in heart rate

13. Which of the following conditions best describes the changes in vasomotor tone with exercise?

	Splanchnic/renal bed resistance	Exercising muscle return	Venous resistance	Venous pressure
a.	Centrally mediated ↑	↓	↑	-
b.	Locally mediated ↑	↓	↑	↑
c.	Centrally mediated ↓	↓	↑	-
d.	Centrally mediated ↑	↓	↓	↓
e.	Locally mediated ↓	↑	↓	↓

14. Which of the following statements best describes the change in myocardial inotropy with exercise?
    a. Contractility increases due to increase in circulating catecholamines and increase in end-diastolic volume (Frank-Starling mechanism)
    b. Contractility increases due to increase in circulating catecholamines, but not an increase in end-diastolic volume (Frank-Starling mechanism)
    c. Contractility decreases due to a paradoxical response to increased circulating catecholamines
    d. Contractility decreases due to a decrease in end-diastolic volume (Frank-Starling mechanism)
    e. Contractility is unchanged with exercise

15. The hemodynamic response to the post-exercise recovery phase is best described in which of the following statements?
    a. Arterial blood pressure transiently rises as systemic vascular resistance increases promptly with cessation of exercise
    b. Arterial blood pressure transiently rises as cardiac output remains elevated while systemic vascular resistance increases
    c. Arterial blood pressure exhibits no change in the recovery period
    d. Arterial blood pressure transiently decreases as systemic vascular resistance increases at a rate proportionally slower than the decrease in cardiac output
    e. Arterial blood pressure transiently decreases as systemic vascular resistance and cardiac output both decrease

Answers

1. **a** Figure 1.1 shows the normal decrease in RA pressure during inspiration, although the amplitude of the pulsations increases—note the increase in the Y-descent. Figure 1.2 shows an abnormal response of RA pressure to inspiration in a patient with constrictive physiology or heart failure. Although the Y-descent is exaggerated, there is no corresponding fall in A- or V-wave height.

2. **c** Kussmaul's sign is a paradoxical rise (or failure to fall) in the height of jugular venous pressure during inspiration. It is commonly seen with congestive heart failure (CHF), constrictive or restrictive physiology, or may be seen in tamponade. Müller's maneuver is defined as inspiration against a closed glottis, imparting negative intrathoracic pressure to the heart, widening the split second sound and augmenting right-sided heart murmurs. Pulsus paradoxus is an exaggerated inspiratory decrease in systemic arterial pressure associated with tamponade physiology. There are no cannon A-waves of atrioventricular dissociation on this tracing. Kussmaul's sign is shown again in Figure 1.9 by the response of the mean RA pressure during inspiration. Duroziez's sign consists of a systolic murmur heard over the FA when it is compressed proximally, and a diastolic murmur when it is compressed distally—this is typical of severe aortic regurgitation.

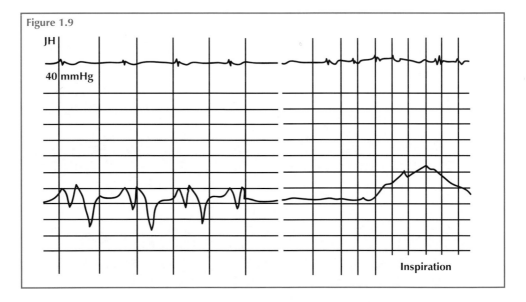

Figure 1.9

3. **e** The RA pressure in a patient with constrictive pericarditis is abnormally elevated with a classic 'M' configuration. The elevated pressure with exaggerated Y-descent after the V-wave is also seen in systolic dysfunction patients. Note the effect of a pacemaker (arrow) on the RA waveform with loss of the A-wave 'x' component.

4. **b** The phasic RA pressure may exceed LA pressure during normal respiration and may greatly exceed LA pressure during Valsalva maneuvers or in the setting of CHF (see Figure 1.10). If the LA and RA pressures are equal, suspect a large atrial septal defect that negates the normal interatrial pressure gradient.

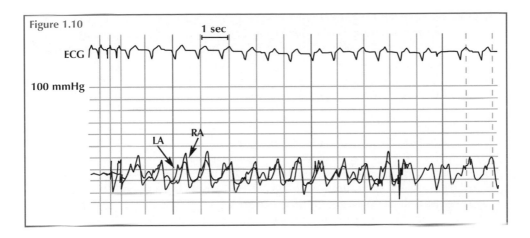

Figure 1.10

5. **1c, 2b, 3a, 4d**

Tracing 1 is (c), a normal central venous or RA pressure waveform. The normal atrial waveform (c) shows two distinct waves and two down slopes. The A-wave is due to atrial systole and follows the p-wave of the ECG. The height of the A-wave depends on atrial contractility and resistance to RV filling. The X-descent follows the A-wave and represents relaxation of the atrium and downward pulling of the tricuspid annulus by RV contraction. The X-descent is interrupted by the C-wave, which is a small positive deflection due to the protrusion of the closed tricuspid valve into the RA. Pressure in the atrium rises after the X-descent from passive filling. The atrial pressure then peaks with the V-wave (representing RV systole). V-wave height is related to atrial compliance and the amount of blood returning to the heart from the periphery. The Y-descent reflects tricuspid valve opening and RA emptying into the RV. The curves are the same in the LA and RA but there is higher mean pressure in the LA, reflecting the higher pressures of the left side of the heart.

Tracing 2 occurs with (b) tricuspid stenosis. Atrial contraction pushing blood through a narrowed tricuspid valve produces an increase in RA pressure and a large A-wave in the RA pressure pulse. The LA waveform demonstrates the same configuration in mitral stenosis.

Tracing 3 is an example of (a) constrictive pericardial disease. The rapid X-descent is absent and the Y-descent is accentuated. The waveform is similar to a square root sign. An attenuated square root sign may be found in cardiac tamponade along with equalization of diastolic pressures in all chambers. Tamponade demonstration increased RA pressure with preserved X-descent but a blunted Y-descent from impeded RA emptying into the RV in early diastole.

Tracing 4 shows waveforms of (d) tricuspid regurgitation. RA pressure is increased due to the regurgitation of blood from the RV in systole producing a large V-wave.

6. **a** The FA pressure is always higher and is delayed in comparison to Ao pressure. The simultaneous FA and LV pressures in the lower panel also show an FA pressure overshoot. If this overshoot is exaggerated after crossing the Ao valve, at least mild Ao stenosis should be suspected.

7. **c** Waveform reflection and summation result in an increase in peak systolic pressure measured at a distance from the central aorta. Severe atherosclerosis or peripheral vascular disease may blunt this femoral overshoot. Ao insufficiency may increase the FA overshoot.

8. **c** The PCW pressure is always delayed relative to its source, the LA. Transit time through the pulmonary veins and capillaries, catheter and tubing account for a 40–120 msec delay. The PCW pressure waveform can be differentiated from the LA waveform by the V-wave peak falling after the down stroke of the LV.

9. **b** Valsalva's maneuver is a common test of the autonomic nervous system that induces an abrupt transient increase in intrathoracic and intra-abdominal pressures. This provokes changes in arterial blood pressure and venous return to the heart. This maneuver was described in 1704 as a method for expelling pus from the middle ear by forced exhalation (straining) with the mouth and nose closed.

10. **a** Valsalva's maneuver increases the minimal and end-diastolic LV pressures, decreases the pulse pressure and increases any LV–Ao gradient in HCM. The normal response to Valsalva's maneuver consists of four phases:
    Phase 1 (initiation) is associated with a transient rise in systemic blood pressure as straining commences. As a rule, Phase 1 cannot be identified at the bedside without invasive monitoring.
    Phase 2 (strain) is accompanied by a perceptible decrease in systemic venous return, blood pressure and pulse pressure and is readily detectable by reflex tachycardia.
    Phase 3 (release) begins promptly, and is associated with an abrupt, transient decrease in blood pressure and in systemic venous return, and is generally not perceived at the bedside without invasive monitoring.
    Phase 4 (recovery) is characterized by an overshoot of systemic arterial pressure and relatively obvious reflex bradycardia. This response provides information about both sympathetic and vagal branches of the autonomic nervous system.

    The Brockenbrough maneuver (purposeful introduction of a premature ventricular beat) normally results in an increased pulse pressure of the subsequent ventricular beat because of an increased diastolic filling period and exaggerated contractile force according to the Frank-Starling mechanism. However, in HCM, the outflow gradient is increased during the post-premature beat, thereby revealing a *decrease* in pulse pressure of the Ao contour. The 'spike and dome' configuration of the Ao pressure waveform may also be accentuated. Ao stenosis is not associated with a dynamic pressure gradient. The Valsalva maneuver is associated with a dynamic pressure gradient.

    The Valsalva maneuver is associated with a decrease in venous return (decreased preload). When coupled with the usual increase in contractile force post-PVC, the (dynamic) gradient is exaggerated.

11. **b** The normal hemodynamic response to exercise is characterized by an increase in cardiac output, a decrease in systemic vascular resistance and a mild increase in mean arterial pressure. The hemodynamic effects of aerobic exercise are summarized in Figure 1.11.

Elie Azrak, James Furgerson, Kenneth LeClerc & Michael D Eisenhauer

Before the onset of exercise, circulatory changes begin with an *anticipatory phase* characterized by an increase in sympathetic nervous system activity, increased heart rate and vasomotor tone. As *aerobic exercise* begins, sympathetic tone increases further and parasympathetic tone decreases, resulting in an increased heart rate, myocardial contractility and arteriolar resistance in the non-exercising vascular beds. Venous return is augmented by an increase in skeletal muscle tone. However, no increase in central venous pressure occurs because of the concomitant increase in myocardial contractility and heart rate. Debate continues regarding changes in LV end-diastolic volume resulting from the augmented venous return, and its subsequent contribution to the inotropic state on the basis of the Frank-Starling mechanism. However, it is generally accepted that the increased myocyte stretch associated with higher end-diastolic volumes contributes to a net increase in contractility during vigorous exercise.

The overall inotropic state is increased with exercise. LV ejection fraction is increased and end-systolic volume is diminished, thereby increasing stroke volume. The increase in stroke volume and heart rate yields an increased cardiac output. In well-trained athletes, the stroke volume may double with maximal exercise, whereas a smaller increase (10–35%) is seen in sedentary patients in response to moderate exercise.

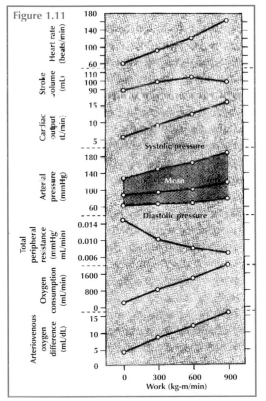

Figure 1.11

Berne RM, Levy MN. Interplay of central and peripheral factors in the control of the circulation. In: Cardiovascular physiology. 7th ed. St. Louis: Mosby-Year Book, 1997: 269–75. (with permission)

Vasomotor changes exhibit a dichotomous response to exercise. With increased levels of circulating catecholamines and sympathetic tone, the vascular resistance to non-exercising territories is increased while resistance to active muscle is decreased due to production of local vasodilator metabolites. The skin is initially in a state of relative vasoconstriction. As core temperature rises, cutaneous vasodilation occurs. The net effect is a decrease in systemic vascular resistance. Because the increase in cardiac output is proportionally greater than the decrease in systemic vascular resistance, the blood pressure tends to increase with exercise. The rise in systolic pressure is greater than the rise in diastolic pressure, so pulse pressure also tends to be exaggerated. The mean arterial pressure shows a mild increase with exercise.

At *peak exertion*, the heart rate and stroke volume reach a plateau (the stroke volume may also decrease slightly), which can sometimes cause a mild decrement in blood pressure at peak exercise. At maximal exercise, the tendency for cutaneous vasodilation is overcome by sympathetic-mediated vasoconstriction that leads to core temperature elevation and a feeling of exhaustion. Other causes of exhaustion include a decrease in pH and lactate accumulation in exercising muscle.

The *recovery phase* of exercise is characterized by a decrease in sympathetic tone with a decrease in heart rate and cardiac output. The systemic vascular resistance slowly decreases in recovery as vasodilating metabolites are cleared. The relatively abrupt drop in cardiac output with the slower increase in systemic vascular resistance yields a tendency for transient hypotension.

12. b Cardiac output rises in normal subjects during exercise. Cardiac output is the product of heart rate and stroke volume, so an increase in cardiac output may be produced by increases in heart rate and/or stroke volume. In the unconditioned subject, the increase in cardiac output is primarily affected by an increase in heart rate, with a small increase in stroke volume. However, in well-conditioned subjects, stroke volume may increase by up to two-fold with maximal exercise.

13. a With exercise, the increase in sympathetic nervous system tone produces an increase in vasomotor tone to non-exercising tissues. This centrally mediated effect is overcome by local metabolites of actively exercising muscle that provoke a decrease in resistance to flow. The net effect is an overall decrease in vasomotor tone with exercise.

14. a Myocardial contractility increases with exercise. This is due primarily to the increase in circulating catecholamines and direct beta stimulation of the myocytes. A second mechanism for enhanced contractility, which is now generally accepted, is increased myocardial stretch via the Frank-Starling mechanism due to augmented venous return with exercise.

15. d A transient decrease in blood pressure is common upon cessation of vigorous exercise. In recovery, systemic vascular resistance increases as vasoactive metabolites are cleared from exercising muscle, and cardiac output decreases as cardiac inotropy and chronotropy decrease. Because the increase in systemic resistance tends to occur more slowly than the decrease in cardiac output, a temporary decrease in blood pressure may occur until these two disparate processes return to pre-exercise levels.

Chapter 2
Aortic Valve Hemodynamics

A 69-year-old man presents with early fatigue, atypical chest pain for 2 years, and two episodes of syncope. A delayed carotid upstroke and systolic murmur are revealed on physical examination. The patient is referred for cardiac catheterization following abnormal echocardiography.

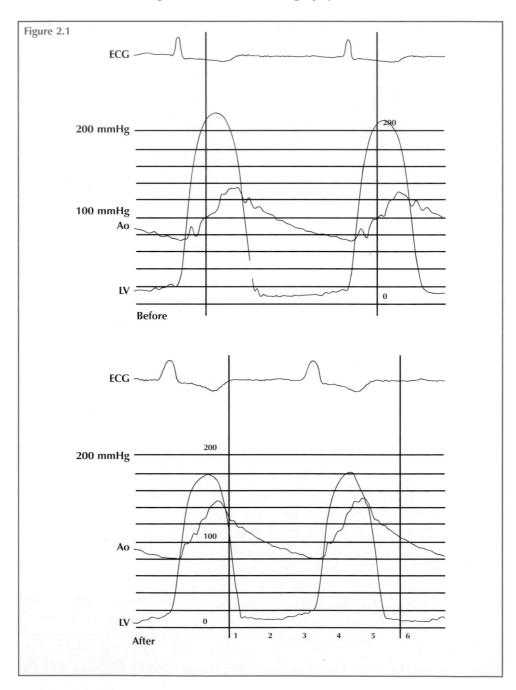

Figure 2.1

The following hemodynamic data are obtained in the catheterization laboratory.

O_2 consumption = 200 mL/min
Hemoglobin (ΔP) = 14 g/dL
Mean gradient = 64 mmHg
Heart rate = 70 bpm
Femoral artery (O_2 sat) = 95%
Pulmonary artery (O_2 sat) = 75%
Peak-peak gradient = 60 mmHg
Peak instantaneous gradient = 140 mmHg
Systolic ejection period (SEP) = 240 msec
Body surface area = 2.0 m²

1. From the available data, what is the most likely explanation for this patient's symptoms?
    a. Hypertrophic cardiomyopathy (HCM)
    b. Degenerative aortic (Ao) stenosis
    c. Congenital bicuspid Ao valve stenosis
    d. Ischemic heart disease
    e. Paroxysmal atrial fibrillation with Ao insufficiency

2. What are the calculated cardiac output (CO) and Ao valve area (AVA)?
    a. CO = 5.25 L/min, AVA = 1.04 cm²
    b. CO = 5.25 L/min; AVA = 0.60 cm²
    c. CO = 5.25 L/min; AVA = 0.88 cm²
    d. CO = 2.67 L/min; AVA = 0.60 cm²
    e. CO = 2.67 L/min; AVA = 0.88 cm²

3. What would the next appropriate step in the management of this patient be?
    a. Surgical consult for Ao valve replacement
    b. Transesophageal echocardiography
    c. Repeat transthoracic echocardiography in 6 months
    d. Exercise Doppler echocardiography
    e. Interventional cardiology consult for balloon-catheter valvuloplasty

4. What potential error is induced if the femoral artery (FA) sheath pressure, rather than the ascending Ao pressure, is used for left ventricular–central Ao (LV–Ao) pressure recordings?
    a. The FA pressure waveform will be dampened, compared to the ascending aorta
    b. The mean Ao valve pressure gradient may be artificially increased
    c. The peak instantaneous Ao valve gradient may be artificially decreased
    d. The calculated AVA (Gorlin's equation) may be artificially increased
    e. A temporal correction to account for pressure wave delay decreases valve area

5. Which sign refers to a rise in Ao pressure during catheter pullback across the Ao valve being associated with severe Ao stenosis?
   a. Carabello's
   b. De Musset's
   c. Traube's
   d. Duroziez's
   e. Müller's

6. When using FA sheath pressure as a comparison to LV pressure in patients with Ao stenosis, what is the effect of using unaligned FA–LV pressure tracings in calculating the gradient and AVA?
   a. Unaligned FA pressures do not influence AVA or gradient
   b. Unaligned FA pressures underestimate AVA and gradient
   c. Unaligned FA pressures overestimate AVA or gradient
   d. Unaligned FA pressures cannot be used to calculate AVA or gradient
   e. Unaligned FA pressures overestimate gradient but underestimate AVA

A 45-year-old man presents with dyspnea on exertion. Physical exam reveals a laterally displaced, hyperdynamic apical impulse and long, decrescendo, blowing diastolic murmur. He was referred for cardiac catheterization after an abnormal transthoracic echocardiogram.

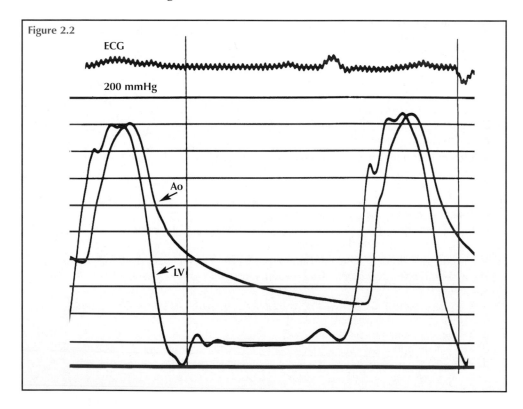

Figure 2.2

ECG

200 mmHg

Ao

LV

The following hemodynamic data are obtained in the catheterization laboratory.

O_2 consumption = 280 mL/min
Hemoglobin = 14 g/dL
Heart rate = 70 bpm
Femoral artery (O_2 sat) = 95%
Pulmonary artery (O_2 sat) = 60%
Angiographic stroke volume = 200 mL

7. Based on the hemodynamic tracing in Figure 2.2, what is the most likely explanation for this patient's symptoms?
    a. Severe Ao stenosis
    b. Hypertrophic obstructive cardiomyopathy
    c. Severe mitral stenosis
    d. Severe Ao regurgitation
    e. Severe pulmonary regurgitation

8. Which of the following is not a potential cause of this patient's condition?
    a. Valine for methionine substitution mutation at position 606 on chromosome 14
    b. Bicuspid Ao valve
    c. Infective endocarditis
    d. Rheumatic fever
    e. Psoriatic arthritis

9. Based on the hemodynamic tracing in Figure 2.2, which clinical presentation is most correct?
    a. Acute, decompensated
    b. Acute, compensated
    c. Chronic, decompensated
    d. Chronic, compensated
    e. Acute Ao dissection

10. This patient's chest radiograph would most likely demonstrate which of the following?
    a. Superior displacement of the left main bronchus
    b. LV enlargement
    c. Right ventricular (RV) enlargement
    d. Normal cardiac silhouette
    e. 'Double density' sign

11. Using the information provided, which index of disease severity can be calculated?
    a. Q_p/Q_s
    b. Regurgitant fraction
    c. Regurgitant orifice
    d. AVA
    e. Mitral valve area

12. If the arterial pressure had been obtained from the Ao position, how might the tracing differ from the one shown in Figure 2.2?
   a. Ao diastolic pressure would be lower
   b. Ao diastolic pressure would be higher
   c. Ao systolic pressure would be lower
   d. Ao systolic pressure would be higher
   e. There would be no difference

13. Auscultation reveals a mid-diastolic apical rumble and no opening snap. This sound would most likely be a(n):
   a. Austin Flint murmur
   b. Carey Coombs murmur
   c. Graham Steell's murmur
   d. Means-Lerman scratch
   e. Still's murmur

A young man had increasing dyspnea on exertion over 3 months. His hypertension is poorly controlled and a new diastolic murmur is present on exam. At catheterization, RV and LV pressures were measured.

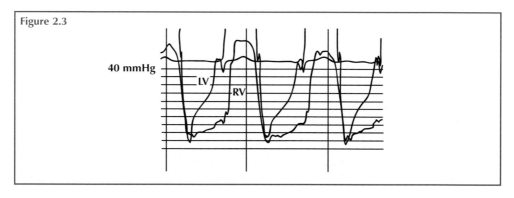

Figure 2.3

40 mmHg

LV

RV

14. Why is the diastolic LV pressure rise greater than the RV diastolic pressure rise?
   a. LV and RV compliance are the same
   b. RV filling is impaired
   c. LV compliance is lower than RV compliance due to rapid LV filling
   d. LV compliance is higher than RV due to rapid LV filling
   e. The LV and RV filling volumes are normal

15. The LV and pulmonary capillary wedge (PCW) pressures of the patient in Question 14 are simultaneously recorded (Figure 2.4). What is the echocardiographic equivalent of this hemodynamic record?
    a. Premature closure of the Ao valve
    b. Severe mitral regurgitation
    c. Flail mitral leaflet
    d. Premature closure of the mitral valve
    e. Premature relaxation of the RV

Figure 2.4

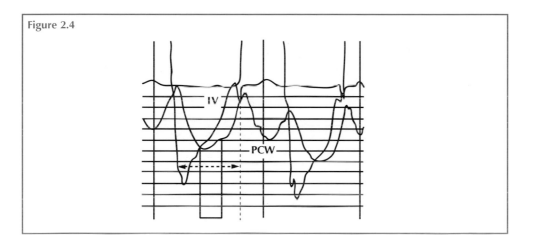

Answers

1. **b** There are three major varieties of adult valvular Ao stenosis: rheumatic, senile-calcific (degenerative), and congenital bicuspid. In degenerative Ao stenosis, calcium accumulates in the pockets of the Ao cusps, which eventually leads to commissural fibrosis. Symptoms usually occur in the seventh decade of life, however they often develop by the fourth or fifth decade in pateints with congenital bicuspid Ao stenosis. There is no delay in the Ao upstroke to suggest a dynamic LV outflow attributable to HCM.

2. **c** $CO = O_2$ consumption / [(Arterial O_2 - Ventricular O_2) x Hb x 1.36* x 10]

   = 200 mL/min / [(0.95 - 0.75) x 14 x 1.36 x 10]

   = 5.25 L/min

   * amount of O_1 carried by 1 g of hemoglobin

   AVA = [CO / (HR x SEP)] / [44.3 x $\sqrt{}$ (Δ P)]

   = [5.25 L/min / (70 beats/min x 0.240 min)] / [†44.3 x $\sqrt{64}$ mmHg]

   = 0.88 cm^2

   (Gorlin's equation)

   †44.3 = empirical constant for aortic and pulmonic valve (mitral valve constant - 37.7)

3. **a** This *symptomatic* patient's Ao stenosis is severe and warrants elective Ao valve replacement surgery without delay.

Severity	Mean gradient (mmHg)	Ao valve area (cm²)
Mild	<25	>1.5
Moderate	25–50	1.0–1.5
Severe	>50	<1.0
Critical	>80	<0.7

In adults with Ao stenosis, the obstruction to LV outflow usually increases gradually over time. LV systolic function is well maintained, accompanied by LV hypertrophy. A large pressure gradient across the Ao valve may be sustained for many years without reducing CO. Congestive symptoms may not appear until LV systolic dysfunction has become severe.

An elevated LV end-diastolic pressure (LVEDP), characteristic of severe Ao stenosis, does not necessarily signify LV dilatation or failure, but more often reflects diminished diastolic compliance of the hypertrophied LV. In this setting, atrial contraction plays a particularly important role, contributing to LV filling and raising LVEDP without producing a concomitant elevation of mean left atrial (LA) pressures or significant pulmonary congestion. The loss of an appropriately timed, vigorous atrial contraction (shown on the first beat of the tracing in Figure 2.1), as seen with atrial fibrillation, junctional rhythm or atrioventricular dissociation, may result in a rapid clinical deterioration.

In the majority of Ao stenosis patients CO is normal at rest, however, it often fails to rise normally with exertion. Significant Ao stenosis exacerbates coexisting mitral regurgitation by increasing the LV–LA pressure gradient. Late in the clinical course, the CO, stroke volume—and therefore the transvalvular pressure gradient—decline. Right heart pressures often rise, resulting in symptomatic congestive heart failure. LV end-diastolic volume usually remains normal until late in the disease with LV chamber dilatation.

4. **b** Due to the elastic properties of the aorta and its major arterial branches, the systolic pressure waveform in the distal FA is often greater than the waveform directly recorded in the ascending aorta. The FA waveform is temporally delayed (see Figure 2.5). Unless a temporal correction is applied the mean transvalvular pressure gradient may be artificially increased, resulting in decreased calculated AVA (more severe stenosis).

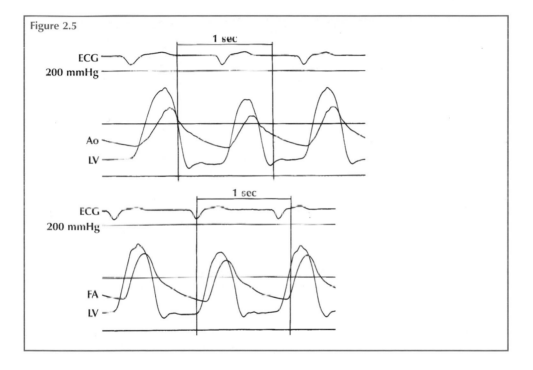

Figure 2.5

If the temporal delay is removed by shifting the FA tracing, the LV gradient may then become smaller than the true gradient (Figure 2.6). The Gorlin equation would therefore be expected to increase the calculated AVA (answer **d**).

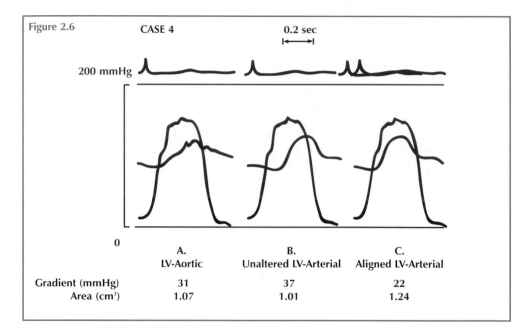

Figure 2.6

CASE 4

0.2 sec

200 mmHg

0

	A. LV-Aortic	B. Unaltered LV-Arterial	C. Aligned LV-Arterial
Gradient (mmHg)	31	37	22
Area (cm³)	1.07	1.01	1.24

5. **a** Carabello first described this sign in 1987, observing that a rise of ≥5 mmHg during single-catheter pullback across the Ao valve was associated with an AVA of ≤0.6 cm². It is believed that partial obstruction of an already narrowed Ao valve orifice by the retrograde catheter, and subsequent relief of that obstruction with pullback, may explain this finding. If suspected, simultaneous dual-transducer measurements of the Ao valve gradient should be performed. Alternatively, a 0.014″ pressure guidewire placed across the Ao valve orifice will not obstruct transvalvular flow while providing a high-fidelity LV pressure recording.

    De Musset's sign (head bobbing with each systolic impulse), Traube's sign (booming systolic and diastolic sounds over the FA), Duroziez's sign (systolic murmur over the FA when it is compressed proximally, and diastolic murmur when it is compressed distally), and Müller's sign (systolic pulsation of the uvula) are all associated with severe Ao regurgitation (AR). Quincke's sign (capillary pulsations) is also seen in severe AR and can be detected by pressing a glass slide on the patient's lip or by transmitting light through the patient's fingertips.

6. **e** The systolic FA pressure peaks after the LV pressure upstroke and is higher than the peak Ao pressure (Figure 2.6) due to summation of peripheral arterial waveforms. Therefore, when using unaligned FA pressure for calculation of AVA, the gradient will be overestimated and the area will be underestimated relative to centrally measured Ao pressure.

7. **d** Two of the earliest symptoms of severe AR are exertional dyspnea and orthopnea. HCM is characterized by a systolic murmur, occasionally with a palpable bisferiens pulse. Similarly, severe Ao stenosis findings include a systolic murmur and delayed, diminished carotid pulsations. In both HCM and severe Ao stenosis, the apical impulse should be sustained and non-displaced. While both mitral stenosis and pulmonary regurgitation cause diastolic murmurs, the hemodynamic tracing is typical of severe AR, with a widened systemic pulse pressure and relatively steep (and then continuing) descent of Ao diastolic pressure throughout diastole.

8. **a** A substitution of valine for methionine on chromosome 14 is associated with hypertrophic cardiomyopathy (HCM). Common causes of AR include a bicuspid Ao valve, infective endocarditis, Ao root disorders (aneurysm, dissection or traumatic disruption) and structural deterioration of prosthetic Ao valves. Uncommon causes include rheumatic disorders (ankylosing spondylitis, rheumatoid arthritis, systemic lupus erythematosus and Takayasu's disease), psoriatic arthritis, Whipple's disease, Crohn's disease and congenital valvular abnormalities.

9. **d** In *chronic* compensated AR the LV adapts to its volume-overload state with both chamber dilatation and myocardial hypertrophy. This adaptive process allows the heart to maintain an effective CO at a normal heart rate, even though 50% or more of the stroke volume returns to the LV during diastole. The large stroke volume ejected by the LV often results in systolic hypertension and contributes significantly to the widened pulse pressure seen in chronic AR. Diastasis (the point at which LV pressure equals LA pressure) occurs in late diastole or early systole.

    In *acute* decompensated AR (Figure 2.7), the LV does not have time to adapt inotropically to the increase in preload. Therefore, an effective CO can only be maintained by increasing the heart rate. Consequently, patients with acute AR are always tachycardic. An increased pulse pressure is rare in this situation because the LV is relatively non-compliant. Tachycardia and limited LV compliance result in smaller regurgitant volumes, smaller stroke volumes and, therefore, lower systolic pressures compared to patients with chronic severe AR. An additional result of the relative non-compliance of the LV is that LV diastolic pressure rises quickly, causing diastasis to occur earlier in diastole. The physical exam correlate demonstrates a diminished or absent S_1, which is seen more commonly in acute severe AR than chronic severe AR.

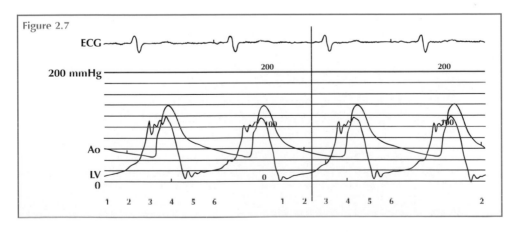

Figure 2.7

10. b Chronic severe AR always results in LV chamber enlargement that may be extreme (*cor bovinum*). Superior displacement of the left mainstem bronchus and the double density sign (overlap of the LA silhouette onto the RA silhouette) are markers of severe LA enlargement, commonly seen in severe mitral stenosis. While RV enlargement can occur in chronic severe AR, it is of minimal clinical or physiologic significance.

11. b Of the options listed, only the regurgitant fraction (RF) can be calculated from the information given. An RF of >55–60% is consistent with severe AR. To calculate the RF the angiographic stroke volume, CO and heart rate must be known.

$$RF = Regurgitant\ Volume\ /\ SV_{angiographic}$$

The angiographic stroke volume (SV) is the total SV (forward SV + regurgitant volume) and is calculated by subtracting the LV end-systolic volume from the LV end-diastolic volume (determined from left ventriculography). The forward SV can be determined by dividing the CO (as determined by the Fick equation) by the heart rate.

The RF can therefore be calculated as follows:

$$RF = (SV_{angiographic} - SV_{forward})\ /\ SV_{angiographic}$$

12. c It is normal to see some degree of systolic pressure amplification in peripheral arteries compared to central Ao pressures. However, in the setting of severe AR it is common to see FA systolic pressures exceed central Ao or LV systolic pressures by 20–50 mmHg. This amplification is thought to be due to the ejection of a very large stroke volume into a relatively compliant arterial system.

13. a The Austin Flint murmur is a mid- to late-diastolic murmur that is common in severe AR. It is believed to be due to rapid regurgitant flow across the mitral valve, whose orifice area is further diminished due to rising LV pressure. Although similar in quality and timing to the murmur of mitral stenosis, the two can often be distinguished by auscultating an opening snap and loud S_1 (which should be present in mitral stenosis and absent in AR). The Carey-Coombs murmur is an early diastolic murmur heard in the setting of active mitral valvulitis due to acute rheumatic fever. The Graham Steell murmur is the murmur of pulmonary regurgitation due to pulmonary hypertension. A Means-Lerman scratch is a mid-systolic sound heard in the setting of thyrotoxicosis. Still's murmur is an innocent, mid-systolic murmur.

14. c *Acute* severe Ao insufficiency results in torrential flow back into the LV and low chamber compliance, which creates a large pressure rise.

Chronic AR requires the LV to adapt and accommodate volume overload state. As described by the Frank-Starling law, the initial response to a moderate increase in LV volume is to increase contractility. However, as the LV enlarges to accommodate the increased volumes, wall stress increases, threatening the increased contractility of the LV. This increase in wall stress triggers a compensatory increase in LV wall thickness, in accordance with Laplace's law, enabling contractility to remain normal. In the setting of volume overload, this hypertrophy occurs eccentrically with sarcomeres replicating primarily in series.

A patient with *chronic compensated* severe AR will have a normal forward stroke volume, ejection fraction and LVEDP even though the end-diastolic volume may be 2–3 times larger than normal. Ultimately, the LV will begin to fail leading to dilatation with a reduction in ejection fraction and an increase in LVEDP.

15. d In acute severe AR the LV does not have the time required to adapt inotropically to accommodate large increases in LV volume and is relatively non-compliant. Consequently, although the LV end-diastolic volume may rise by <2 times the normal level, the LVEDP will rise exponentially.

Patients with acute severe AR exhibit reduced forward stroke volumes, a narrowed pulse pressure, smaller LV volumes and faster heart rates compared to patients with a similar severity of AR that has developed chronically.

Premature closure of the mitral valve is represented by early LV–PCW pressure crossover

Symptomatic, severe AR is a clear indication for surgery. However, it is not always clear how to manage asymptomatic patients with chronic severe AR. Natural history studies have demonstrated that the best predictor of long-term survival in patients with severe AR is preoperative LV function. Consequently, many physicians recommend surgical referral when the ejection fraction falls to less than 'normal', and/or when the LV end systolic diameter exceeds 50 mm.

Chapter 3
Mitral Valve Hemodynamics

A 49-year-old woman has progressive dyspnea on exertion. As a child she recalls a prolonged 'febrile' illness associated with joint ache and a rash. A heart murmur was found on high school physical exam. Her echocardiogram suggests mitral valve disease. Cardiac catheterization revealed the following hemodynamic tracing (Figure 3.1).

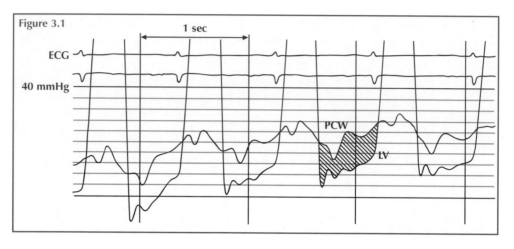

Figure 3.1

1. Based on the hemodynamics (Figure 3.1), one might conclude that this patient most likely has:
   a. Mitral regurgitation (MR)
   b. Mitral stenosis (MS) with an estimated valve gradient of 25 mmHg
   c. Poor quality pulmonary capillary wedge (PCW) pressure—one cannot assess the exact gradient
   d. Diastolic dysfunction
   e. Normal V-wave

In the same patient as in Question 1, the PCW and direct left atrial (LA) pressures (obtained using transseptal technique) are compared (Figure 3.2).

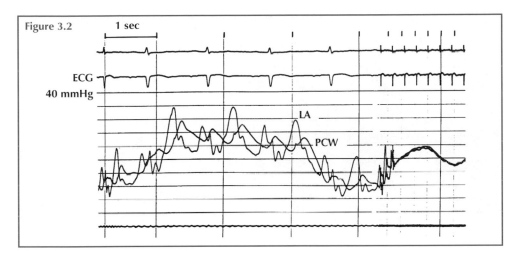

2. Based on these tracings (Figure 3.2), which statement is true?
   a. The fidelity of the PCW pressure wave is equal to the LA pressure wave
   b. The A-wave of the LA is equal to that of the PCW
   c. The V-wave of the LA is less than that of the PCW
   d. The mean pressures of the PCW and LA are equal
   e. Either pressure tracing can be used to assess MS

The direct LA pressure, measured using the transseptal approach, and the left ventricular (LV) pressures are now recorded (Figure 3.3).

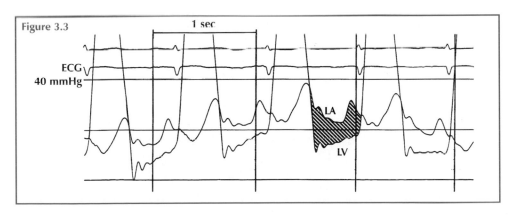

3. Regarding the hemodynamics in Figure 3.3, which of the following statements is true?
   a. The rhythm is atrial fibrillation
   b. The mean LA–LV gradient is approximately 14 mmHg
   c. The LA A-wave is larger than the V-wave
   d. There is severe MR
   e. Mitral balloon valvuloplasty is contraindicated

Mitral balloon valvuloplasty is performed (Figure 3.4) and the following hemodynamics are recorded (Figure 3.5).

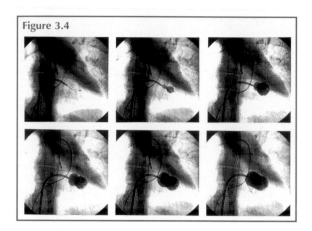

Figure 3.4

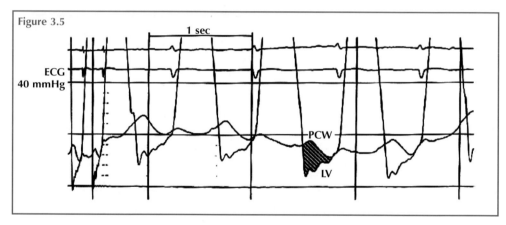

Figure 3.5

4. Which of the following statements is true with regard to Figures 3.4 and 3.5?
   a. There is no residual significant gradient
   b. There is severe MR
   c. There may be a significant mitral gradient
   d. The procedure is finished
   e. The PCW is a reliable tracing to gauge mitral gradients in this patient

Following measurement of direct LA pressure, the following hemodynamics were recorded (Figure 3.6).

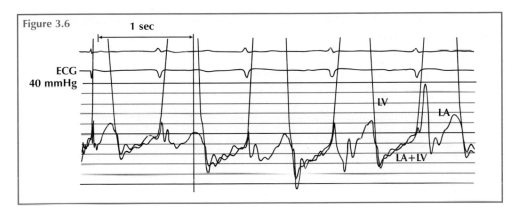

Figure 3.6

5. Which of the following statements is true?
   a. There is no residual significant gradient
   b. There is severe MR
   c. There may be a significant mitral gradient
   d. The procedure is not finished
   e. The PCW is a reliable tracing to gauge mitral gradients in this patient

A 65-year-old man with a remote history of inferior myocardial infarction presents with progressive dyspnea, fatigue and decreased exercise tolerance over the last year. Physical exam reveals an holosystolic murmur radiating to the axilla, laterally displaced apical impulse and basilar rales. He is referred for cardiac catheterization following echocardiography. Hemodynamic data are shown in Figure 3.7.

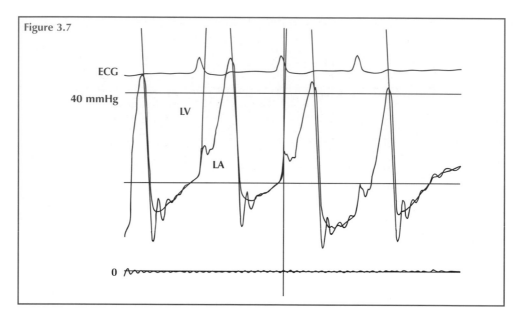

Figure 3.7

6. Based on the hemodynamic tracing in Figure 3.7, which is the most likely cause of his symptoms?
    a. Symptomatic coronary artery disease (CAD)
    b. Aortic stenosis
    c. MS
    d. MR
    e. Hypertrophic obstructive cardiomyopathy

7. What finding on the hemodynamic tracing (Figure 3.7) is classically seen with the diagnosis in this patient?
    a. Giant A-waves
    b. Rapid X-descent
    c. Large V-waves with prolonged Y-descent
    d. Giant V-waves with rapid Y-descent
    e. Early diastolic LA–LV gradient with prolonged X-descent

8. **What is the rhythm shown in Figure 3.7?**
    a. Normal sinus rhythm
    b. Multifocal atrial tachycardia
    c. Atrial fibrillation
    d. Atrial flutter
    e. Junctional or idioventricular rhythm

9. **In the LA pressure tracing on Figure 3.7, using the QRS pattern as the starting point, identify the waveform deflections.**
    a. A-wave, V-wave
    b. V-wave, A-wave
    c. C-wave, V-wave
    d. V-wave, C-wave
    e. Y-descent, A-wave

10. **Based on the patient's clinical presentation and hemodynamic tracing in Figure 3.7, which statement is most accurate? The LA is likely to be:**
    a. Small and compliant
    b. Small and non-compliant
    c. Small and semi-compliant
    d. Large and compliant
    e. Large and non-compliant

11. **Based on the hemodynamic tracing in Figure 3.7, which of the following diagnoses can be excluded?**
    a. Ventricular septal defect
    b. MS
    c. Rheumatic heart disease involving the LA wall
    d. Pericardial constriction
    e. Coronary artery disease

12. **Echocardiography reveals severe MR secondary to postero-medial papillary muscle dysfunction, and an LV ejection fraction (LVEF) of 50%. What is your therapeutic recommendation?**
    a. Repeat an ECG in 6 months and continue endocarditis prophylaxis
    b. Increase afterload-reducing agents (ACE inhibitors)
    c. Add preload-reducing agents (nitroglycerin)
    d. Refer for surgical mitral valve repair or replacement
    e. Add inotropic agents (digoxin)

LA and LV pressures are measured in a patient with MS (Figure 3.8).

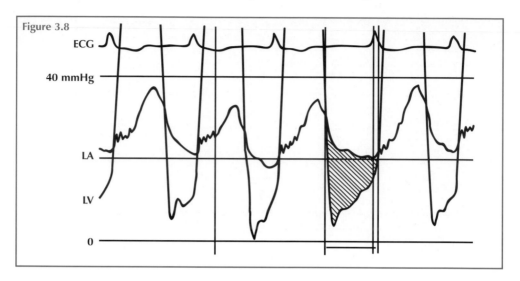

Figure 3.8

13. Based on Figure 3.8, the V-wave indicates the presence of severe MR.
    a. True
    b. False

14. Which of the following conditions does not reduce compliance in the LA?
    a. Rheumatic fever
    b. Cardiac surgery
    c. Systemic lupus erythematosus
    d. Pericarditis
    e. Chronic MR

Answers

1. **c** The tracing demonstrates a poor quality PCW pressure that does not clearly delineate the A-wave or the V-wave. The gradient cannot be determined precisely based on the quality of the tracing. However, the estimate of the valve gradient from this tracing would not exceed 16 mmHg. The patient probably does not have significant MR since there is no V-wave. The precise degree of MS cannot be determined from the tracings. Diastolic dysfunction is not present, as shown by the normal increasing rise of LV diastolic pressure across the diastolic period. A normal V-wave with a PCW pressure wave artifact is a remote possibility but inconsistent with the physical exam.

2. **d** The two mean pressures are the same, although the fidelity of the LA waveform is much better than that of the PCW pressure waveform. The largest and most predominant LA waveform is that of the V-wave. The LA V-wave is larger than that of the PCW pressure in this tracing. If both the fidelity and quality of the tracings were the same, either tracing could be used to assess MS. However, this is *not* the case here.

3. **b** The mean LA–LV pressure gradient is approximately 14 mmHg, which can be estimated by counting the number of 4 mmHg divisions across the pressure waveform. An estimation of the V-wave area (MVA) can be made using the quick (Hakki) formula or (MVA = cardiac output divided by the square root of the mean gradient). This quick formula does not apply in heart rates >100 or <60 beats/minute. The V-wave is larger than the A-wave. The patient is not in atrial fibrillation due to the fact that there is an A-wave on the LA tracing despite no visible P-wave on the ECG. A large V-wave alone does not necessarily indicate severe MR. Mitral balloon valvuloplasty is indicated if ECG and patient findings are suitable.

4. **c** Based on the poor quality of the PCW pressure and the continued gradient across diastole, there may be a significant mitral gradient using this flawed technique. MR is not likely to be severe. The V-wave is small. The procedure is not complete until we further assess whether this is an accurate mitral gradient or not, as the PCW is not a reliable tracing to gauge mitral gradients in this patient.

5. **a** Based on direct LA and LV tracings, there is no significant gradient left after the valvuloplasty procedure. The procedure is therefore finished. There is no significant V-wave, suggesting MR occurred. There is little potential for erroneous gradient calculations unless major zeroing errors have occurred. The PCW pressure is not a reliable tracing to gauge mitral gradients in this patient.

   Pressure waveforms used in the calculation of MS must be reliable and of such quality that a pressure gradient can be determined both before and after interventions. Given the damped and poor quality phasic tracing of the PCW pressure, LA pressure should be used both before and after a balloon valvuloplasty procedure to assess the quality of the results. Erroneous assumptions regarding the presence or absence of gradients can be made if one relies on PCW pressure tracings without good fidelity tracings. Calculation of MVAs can be made with the Gorlin formula or the Hakki formula with appropriate precautions based on heart rate.

6. **d** The diagnosis of severe MR is supported by the history, physical exam and hemodynamic tracing, which reveal increased LA pressure and characteristic giant V-waves. MS can also be associated with large V-waves, reflecting a low compliance (stiff) chamber. MS combined with MR will also demonstrate a diastolic gradient. The V-wave of MS tracings does not necessarily indicate significant MR. Another clue in MS is the early LA–LV diastolic gradient with prolonged X- and Y-descents, reflecting obstructed atrial outflow. In this tracing, the LA and LV diastolic pressures are equal, and the Y-descent is identical to the downslope of early LV diastole, thereby demonstrating no significant obstruction to atrial outflow. Symptomatic CAD can present as progressive dyspnea and fatigue, and may even cause acute MR from papillary muscle dysfunction secondary to ischemia or infarction. This patient's symptoms have been insidious in onset, with evidence of a dilated LV by echocardiography. The MR murmur on exam is consistent with uncompensated chronic severe MR. Although associated with elevated LV diastolic pressures, hypertrophic obstructive cardiomyopathy cannot be diagnosed on the findings provided.

Common causes of MR include mitral leaflet and/or subchordal apparatus malformation, papillary muscle dysfunction and loss of mitral valvular annulus geometry. Common etiologies of MR include CAD, rheumatic heart disease, infective endocarditis, mitral valve prolapse syndrome and viral cardiomyopathies.

7. **d** Giant V-waves are defined as V-waves with an amplitude of more than twice the mean LA or PCW pressure. Giant V-waves are most likely to occur in acute MR, but can occur whenever there is reduced LA compliance and increased volume, as seen with ventricular septal defect or MS. Severe MR is associated with a rapid Y-descent with no early LA–LV diastolic gradient, thereby representing unobstructed LA outflow. Isolated MS, or mixed MS and MR, is associated with both a diastolic gradient and prolonged Y-descent representing obstructed LA outflow.

8. **c** The absence of A-waves and the irregularly irregular rhythm are consistent with atrial fibrillation. Both sinus rhythm and atrial flutter are associated with identifiable A-waves. Although A-waves are absent with idioventricular or junctional rhythms, these rhythms are usually regular, or have identifiable retrograde activation of the atria (with a P-wave on ECG or A-wave on pressure recording).

9. **c** The C-wave represents the onset of ventricular contraction and occurs just inside the upstroke of the LV pressure tracing. In normal sinus rhythm, the C-wave is a small positive deflection often within the X-descent and is only rarely seen. In this patient, the V-wave results from the LV systolic regurgitant volume filling a non-compliant LA. With simultaneous LA/LV pressure tracings, the peak V-wave occurs just inside the downslope of the LV pressure tracing. In simultaneous PCW/LV pressure tracings, there is a 40–120 msec pressure transmission delay, so the peak V-wave is recorded as occurring just after the rapid downslope of the LV tracing in early diastole (see Figure 3.9). There is no A-wave because the patient is in atrial fibrillation.

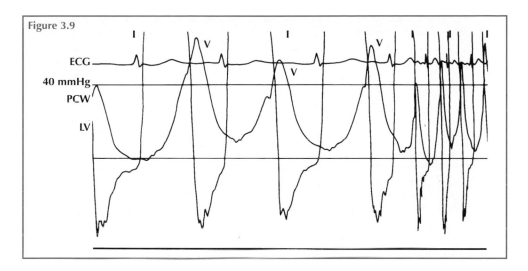

Figure 3.9

10. e The patient presents with insidious onset of dyspnea, fatigue and decreased exercise tolerance over the previous year. This is consistent with decompensated severe chronic MR with a large LA that has become maximally dilated and cannot accommodate any further increase in volume without subsequent increase in LA pressure.

MR provides the LV with two outlets through both the aortic and mitral valves. The regurgitant flow results in decreased forward cardiac output with a portion going into the LA, which subsequently returns to increase left heart volume. The ability to compensate for the volume overload and the associated hemodynamic consequences depends on both LA and LV compliance.

11. b This pressure tracing does not support the diagnosis of MS, given an absence of an early diastolic LA–LV gradient and the presence of a rapid Y-descent consistent with unobstructed LA outflow. V-waves are caused by the LA pressure-volume relationship and are most prominent in a non-compliant LA. Other conditions that have large V-waves include ventricular septal defect, MS (with LA–LV gradient), non-compliant LA secondary to rheumatic heart disease, pericardial constriction (although in this patient the LV waveform is not consistent with pericardial constraint), or other post-operative or inflammatory changes.

12. d Treatment goals for acute severe MR include immediate afterload reduction, and the addition of inotropic agents if the patient is hypotensive. An intra-aortic balloon pump also reduces afterload and increases forward systemic arterial flow. Acute MR is often poorly tolerated, and many patients require emergency mitral valve repair or replacement. Even in the presence of severe LV systolic dysfunction, the LVEF can appear to be preserved as a result of increased preload and favorable afterload reduction resulting from the MR itself.

After mitral valve surgery, MR patients with preserved LV size and function have a greater chance of retaining a normal LV function. Symptomatic patients (NYHA class III–IV) with severe MR should be directly referred for mitral valve repair or replacement. Asymptomatic patients with severe MR, a dilated LV (>45 mm end-systole) and/or a low normal EF (<55–60%) should also be referred to surgery. The development of atrial fibrillation or secondary pulmonary hypertension is also an indication for mitral valve surgery, even in asymptomatic patients. Endocarditis prophylaxis is advised for all patients with significant MR.

Chronic MR patients may remain asymptomatic for years. Both the LA and LV dilate in order to accommodate the volume-overloaded state. The LA remodels, and the LV hypertrophies by increasing the number of new sarcomeres in a serial pattern (as opposed to the parallel pattern seen with hypertensive hypertrophy). The degree of hypertrophy continues as the LV dilatation progresses, such that the ratio of LV mass to end-diastolic volume remains constant. The length of the individual myocardial fibers is increased, thereby allowing the LV chamber to dilate and accept the increased volume without significant changes in intracavitary pressure. In the compensated state, cardiac output is maintained by an increased total stroke volume resulting from an increased LV preload. Invasive hemodynamics may be misleading in some patients—LA pressures may be normal and large V-waves may be absent. When further cavitary dilation is not possible the LV and LA become less compliant, resulting in abnormal hemodynamics with systolic dysfunction late in the patient's course. Once symptoms develop, or there is reduced LV systolic function (end-systolic diameter >45 mm or LVEF <55%), surgery should be considered.

Acute MR patients present with dyspnea and pulmonary congestion, secondary to a sudden increase in LA and LV end-diastolic pressures (LVEDP) from uncompensated volume overload. The LV may dilate acutely in the absence of eccentric hypertrophy, resulting in reduced stroke volume and decreased forward output. The decrease in cardiac output increases LVEDP, and could lead to cardiogenic shock. The LA is less compliant in the acute course, resulting in increased LA pressures with characteristic giant V-waves on the hemodynamic tracings, and increased pulmonary pressures that may lead to pulmonary edema.

13. b The V-wave cannot be used alone to characterize MR in the absence of clinical findings since the major factor for generating V-waves is LA compliance. According to the compliance curves (Figure 3.10), any condition that reduces compliance can result in a disproportionatly large V-wave subsequent to even a minor change in regurgitant volume.

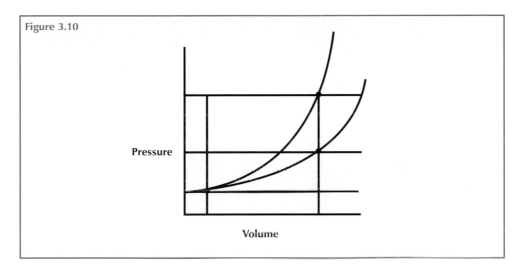

Figure 3.10

Pressure

Volume

14. e Chronic exposure to increased flow and pressure causes a gradual increase in compliance of the chamber. Any acute or chronic inflammatory conditions, including post-surgery inflammation, generally reduce compliance and may result in a large V-wave without true MR.

Chapter 4
Tricuspid Valve Hemodynamics

A 70-year-old woman presents with an acute onset of retrosternal chest pain and shortness of breath. She had rheumatic fever and mitral regurgitation requiring a Starr-Edwards valve in the mitral position 30 years ago. Echocardiography shows a normal functioning valve prosthesis with bi-atrial and right ventricular (RV) enlargement. She reports an intermittent febrile illness.

Her blood pressure was 130/70 mmHg; pulse was irregular at 60 bpm. The jugular venous pressure was 5 cm with prominent V-waves. Cardiac auscultation revealed a prominent metallic click with a grade II/VI systolic murmur at the left sternal border, which varied with respiration. Pre-catheterization laboratory values were normal except for a troponin I of 7.5. The electrocardiogram (ECG) showed atrial fibrillation without ST or T-wave abnormalities.

The following hemodynamic tracing of the right atrial (RA) pressure (Figure 4.1) was obtained during right heart catheterization performed with a balloon-tipped Swan-Ganz catheter.

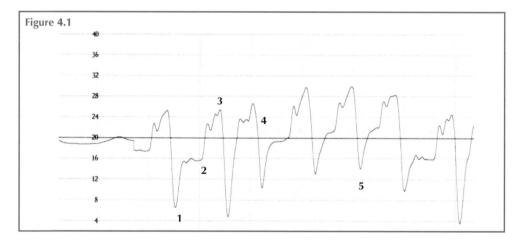

Figure 4.1

1. In the hemodynamic tracing in Figure 4.1, waveform #3 represents:
   a. Prominent A-wave of mitral valve dysfunction
   b. Prominent V-wave due to high left ventricular (LV) pressure
   c. Prominent A-wave of tricuspid valve regurgitation
   d. Prominent V-wave of tricuspid valve regurgitation
   e. Respiratory artifact

2. The most likely cause of the condition in this patient is:
   a. Carcinoid heart disease
   b. Rheumatic heart
   c. RV infarction
   d. Infective endocarditis
   e. Myxomatous degeneration (tricuspid valve prolapse)

3. The V-wave on the RA tracing can be confirmed temporally by which component of the ECG?
    a. The P-wave
    b. The end of the QRS complex
    c. The T-wave
    d. The QT segment
    e. The PR segment

4. Which of the following best explains the differences between the Y-descents labeled #1 and #5?
    a. Atrial fibrillation
    b. Transient ischemia
    c. Normal respiration
    d. Kussmaul's sign
    e. Restoration of normal sinus rhythm

A 72-year-old woman with rheumatoid arthritis and interstitial lung disease is referred for evaluation of shortness of breath and atypical chest pain. She has no prior diagnosis of heart disease. Your evaluation includes right heart catheterization as shown in Figure 4.2.

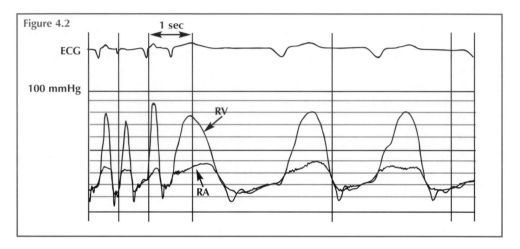

Figure 4.2

5. The condition illustrated in the tracing on Figure 4.2 shows which of the following?
   a. Rapid X-descent
   b. Delayed Y-descent
   c. Prominent or peaked A-wave
   d. Minimized V-wave
   e. Ventricularization of V-wave

6. Which of the following maneuvers will increase the murmur intensity and hemodynamic findings of this condition?
   a. Valsalva
   b. Müller
   c. Handgrip
   d. Standing from a seated position
   e. Intravenous nitroglycerin

7. In the absence of other cardiac pathology, associated findings in this disorder include all of the following except:
   a. Pulmonary congestion
   b. Overshoot of the murmur after release of Valsalva maneuver
   c. Atrial fibrillation
   d. Rapid Y-descent of venous pulsations
   e. Systolic pulsations of an enlarged and tender liver

8. **Etiologies for this condition include all of the following except:**
   a. RV myocardial infarction
   b. Severe pulmonary vascular disease
   c. Hypothyroidism
   d. Rheumatic heart disease
   e. Carcinoid heart disease

9. **Which of the following would not be an expected part of this patient's management?**
   a. Treatment of other coexistent valvular disease
   b. Ring annuloplasty, if symptomatic and pulmonary hypertension is documented
   c. β-Blocker therapy, with target heart rate ≤60 bpm
   d. Conservative management, if the patient is asymptomatic
   e. Diuresis

A 47-year-old female with atrial fibrillation is referred for a second opinion. Her evaluation included right heart catheterization. The hemodynamic tracings are shown in Figure 4.3.

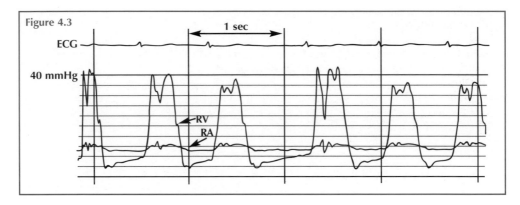

Figure 4.3

10. Which clinical symptom(s) would this woman likely report?
    a. Hemoptysis
    b. Paroxysmal nocturnal dyspnea
    c. Weight loss
    d. Lower extremity edema
    e. Chest pain

11. Associated physical exam findings include all of the following except:
    a. Prominent venous A-wave pulsation
    b. Diastolic murmur that decreases with inspiration
    c. Diastolic murmur that increases with inspiration
    d. Ascites
    e. Diastolic murmur that decreases with passive leg raising

12. Maneuvers that could accentuate the pressure gradient shown include all of the following except:
    a. Deep inspiration
    b. Rapid intravenous fluid bolus
    c. Valsalva maneuver
    d. Dynamic exercise
    e. Amyl nitrite inhalation

13. **Potential underlying etiologies of this woman's disorder include all of the following except:**
    a. Rheumatic valvular disease
    b. Prosthetic valve malfunction
    c. Vegetations of the tricuspid valve
    d. RA myxoma
    e. Carcinoid heart disease

14. **Initial clinical management of this condition may include:**
    a. Diuresis
    b. Inotropic therapy
    c. Heart transplantation
    d. Progressive exercise program
    e. Balloon valvotomy

Answers

1. **d** Tricuspid regurgitation (TR) is associated with large right-sided V-waves, which can be seen on inspection of the venous pulse in the neck. The regurgitant impulse may be palpable over the RA and liver. The RV may be hyperdynamic. The murmur of TR is holosystolic and increases with inspiration. With RV dysfunction, an S_3 gallop may be present.

    The primary hemodynamic features of TR are the prominent V-wave and the progressive rise in RA pressure throughout RV systole. This V-wave prominence may take on the form of an RV pressure wave in extreme cases. However, a prominent V-wave may not always be evident, even in cases of moderate to severe TR. A prominent V-wave of >12 mmHg has a low positive predictive value (62%) for the presence of moderate to severe TR. A high negative predictive value (89%) suggests that the absence of a V-wave of >12 mmHg is actually better at excluding moderate or severe TR.

    Individuals with TR are generally asymptomatic, with the underlying etiologic cause of the TR (i.e. RV failure, mitral stenosis [MS]) having far greater impact on their clinical status and management. Manifestations of TR reflect decreased cardiac output (CO) with venous congestion (jugular venous distention, hepatic congestion leading to ascites), weakness and fatigue. Pertinent exam findings include prominent V-wave and rapid Y-descent of venous pulsations, an holosystolic murmur that increases with inspiration (Carvallo's sign), an irregular rhythm of atrial fibrillation and (if severe) manifestations of RV failure.

    Clinical management ranges from no specific therapy to surgical replacement of the incompetent valve. Most often, medical management is directed at the precipitating condition. If severe TR persists, the preferred surgical approach is suture or ring annuloplasty with total valve replacement remaining a secondary option only.

2. **d** TR is a common valvular abnormality, which results from backflow of blood from the RV into the RA during systole. Primary TR occurs principally as a result of endocarditis. However, other causes include rheumatic disease, Ebstein's anomaly, Marfan's syndrome, carcinoid heart disease and tricuspid valve prolapse. Secondary TR occurs when the tricuspid valve annulus is dilated as in cases of pulmonary hypertension, pulmonic stenosis or RV infarction.

3. **c**

4. **c** The Y-descent increases (steeper slope) during inspiration (#1) and decreases over the respiratory cycle, becoming more shallow at the end of expiration (#5). Transmitted negative intrathoracic pressures during inspiration cause the RV diastolic pressures to be reduced in comparison to expiration, when intrathoracic pressures are neutral. Hence true central venous (filling) pressures are more accurately determined on expiration. The heights of the A- and V-waves are most often determined by the compliance of the atria and ventricles. In this patient, the severity of the TR influences the size and speed of the V-wave and Y-descent.

5. **e** Figure 4.2 reveals both TR and severe pulmonary hypertension. The two key features are the prominent V-wave and the progressive rise in RA pressure throughout RV systole. In its most severe form, it may take the appearance of an RV pressure wave form (ventricularization): since the V-wave is elevated, the associated Y-descent (not the X-descent) would be accentuated. A peaked A-wave would be seen in tricuspid stenosis (TS). A labeled generic atrial waveform is shown in Figure 4.4.

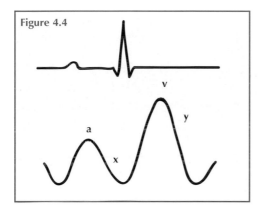

Figure 4.4

Simultaneous measurement of RA and ventricular pressures shows equilibration during diastole (assuming no coexistent TS) with RA pressure increasing further during systole as the regurgitant volume fills the right atrium.

In general, TR is well tolerated until the onset of pulmonary hypertension. Medical therapy includes a low sodium diet and fluid restriction. Diuretics may be used for edema, and digoxin prescribed for RV dysfunction. Although pulmonary pressures respond poorly to medical therapy, nitrates and calcium channel blockers have been used. In cases of coexisting LV dysfunction, afterload reduction is suggested. Symptomatic TR may also be treated with annuloplasty. In the case of endocarditis or Ebstein's anomaly, tricuspid valve repair or replacement is warranted, although the risk of thrombosis for mechanical valves in this position is high.

From a variety of cardiac and pulmonary processes, RV failure is the predominant etiologic cause of TR rather than intrinsic abnormalities of the tricuspid valve. RV failure and dilatation from pulmonary hypertension lead to a dilated tricuspid valve annulus and valvular incompetence. More common underlying causes of TR include pulmonary parenchymal or vascular disease, RV infarction, LV papillary muscle dysfunction and other types of cardiomyopathies. Additional, but less frequent, causes of TR include primary rheumatic valvular disease, endocarditis, Ebstein's anomaly, carcinoid heart disease and trauma.

6. **b** Since this is a right-sided valve disorder, maneuvers that increase transvalvular flow would be expected to enhance the murmur of TR. These would include inspiration (Carvallo's sign), Muller maneuver (forced inspiration against a closed glottis), passive leg raising, dynamic exercise (not handgrip) and hepatic compression. Phase II (strain phase) of the Valsalva maneuver is associated with a decreased systemic venous return, as is IV nitroglycerin administration. Similarly, standing from a seated position reduces venous return to the right heart, and would decrease the systolic murmur of TR.

7. **a** Clinical findings of a right-sided abnormality, such as pure TR, are reflected by the consequences of the valvulopathy. Common findings include RV failure, pulmonary hypertension and venous congestion (ascites and peripheral edema predominate). Atrial fibrillation is a common finding. Systolic hepatic pulsations may be palpable initially, but may disappear in chronic TR with congestive cirrhosis, in which the liver may become firm and non-tender. The transient increase in trans-tricuspid flow after release of Valsalva straining (Phases III and IV) accentuates the pansystolic murmur of TR, but may be present for only the first 2 or 3 cycles following release. As noted previously, a rapid Y-descent after the heightened V-wave might be detected on examination of jugular venous pulsations. Pulmonary congestion is a finding indicative of left heart failure.

8. **c** There is no relationship between hypothyroidism and TR, although TR may be a presenting manifestation of thyrotoxicosis. Answers a, b, d and e are all potential etiologies of TR. Right-sided heart failure may be intensified in the presence of severe pulmonary hypertension, thereby causing dilatation of the RV and tricuspid valve annulus with worsening TR.

9. **c** Management of TR is dictated by its severity and concomitant symptoms, and/or the presence of moderate to severe pulmonary hypertension. Initial management should address coexistent valvular disease (such as MS), which may be more influential on clinical status, thereby indirectly exacerbating the TR. Benefit may be obtained by reducing RV volume overload through the judicious use of diuretics. In the setting of symptoms attributable to TR and significant pulmonary hypertension (pulmonary artery systolic [PAS] pressure >60 mmHg), surgical repair with suture or ring annuloplasty is a preferred approach, with valve replacement being a second option.

10. **d** This tracing demonstrates TS. The clinical manifestations of significant TS reflect increased RA pressures. Therefore, symptoms such as lower extremity edema and weight gain (particularly if ascites is coexistent) are likely to be reported. Symptoms reflective of left heart failure, such as paroxysmal nocturnal dyspnea, are likely to be absent. Hemoptysis may be associated with mitral valve stenosis, but is not usually associated with TS.

    TS is most often caused by rheumatic heart disease (RHD). Other conditions such as RA tumors involving the valve leaflets, endocarditic vegetations, prosthetic valve malfunction, congenital defects, carcinoid heart disease, Fabry's disease and Whipple's disease are other less common etiologies. In RHD, the patient's clinical symptoms and management are more likely to be determined by left-sided valve involvement, such as MS. Nonetheless, TS may progress to hemodynamic and clinical significance.

11. **b** The murmur of a stenotic atrioventricular valve (either MS or TS) is predominantly diastolic, but only TS would be accentuated with the increased blood flow return to the more compliant RV produced with inspiration. Passive leg-raising increases systemic venous return. The significant increase in central venous pressure resulting from TS may cause hepatic congestion and ascites.

12. **c** The tricuspid valve gradient is increased with any maneuver that increases flow into the right heart and across the tricuspid valve. Of the maneuvers listed, all would increase filling (and flow) of the right heart except the Valsalva maneuver. During phase II (straining phase) of the Valsalva maneuver, systemic venous return declines, and filling of the right heart, and then the left heart, is reduced. Borderline gradients can be further clarified

with maneuvers that increase transvalvular flow such as inspiration, rapid infusion of fluid, dynamic exercise or atropine. Amyl nitrite inhalation produces marked vasodilation, resulting in the first 30 seconds in a reduction of systemic arterial pressure, and 30–60 seconds later in a reflex tachycardia, followed in turn by a reflex increase in CO, blood flow velocity and heart rate. The increase in CO augments the diastolic murmurs of MS, TS and pulmonic regurgitation as well as the systolic murmur of TR.

13. e While carcinoid heart disease classically involves right heart structures and may involve the tricuspid valve specifically, it is more likely to produce TR rather than stenosis. Answers a–d may all be associated with clinically significant obstruction to flow from the RA to the RV.

14. a Initial management should focus on reducing the elevated right-sided pressure and volume. This can be accomplished with diuresis and sodium restriction. Inotropic therapy and an evaluation for heart transplantation are not initially indicated. Regular exercise is not expected to dramatically improve the clinical situation. Exercise is not discouraged, but is likely to be limited by the severity of the symptoms. This is particularly true if concomitant MS is present.

In situations where TS is predominant, the clinical presentation and exam findings reflect an increased venous pressure (e.g. prominent jugular venous A-waves, ascites, lower extremity edema and fatigue). Clinical management is dictated by the patient's symptoms, underlying etiology of the TS and concomitant valvular disease. Invasive management includes surgical commissurotomy, balloon valvuloplasty or surgical replacement (or removal) of the tricuspid valve. The development of a diastolic RA/RV mean pressure gradient of 5 mmHg or valve area of ≤ 2.0 cm^2 is usually an indication for intervention

Chapter 5
Pulmonary Valve Hemodynamics

A 19-year-old woman has an ejection systolic murmur along the upper left sternal border, which was detected during routine physical examination. She is asymptomatic and not cyanotic. The pressure tracings from right heart catheterization are shown in Figure 5.1.

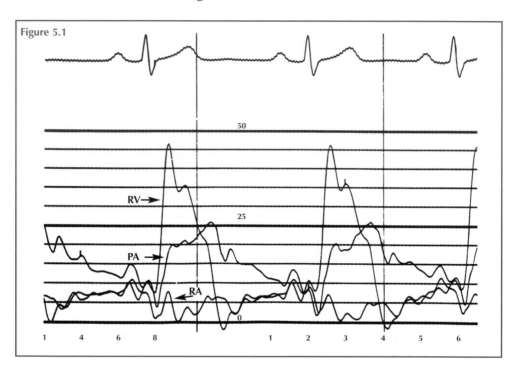

Figure 5.1

1. What is the most likely diagnosis based on Figure 5.1?
    a. Ventricular septal defect (VSD) and pulmonary stenosis (PS)
    b. Tetralogy of Fallot
    c. Atrial septal defect (ASD)
    d. PS
    e. Idiopathic dilation of the pulmonary artery (PA) with pulmonary insufficiency

2. All of the following statements regarding the systolic gradient in Figure 5.1 are false except:
    a. In severe PS, the PA pressure tracing retains its pulsatile configuration despite the reduction in mean pressure
    b. Gorlin's formula can be used to estimate the severity of the associated infundibular stenosis
    c. Heart rate is the most important correlate with the gradient across the pulmonary valve
    d. In severe PS, the stroke volume increases significantly during exercise, which increases the gradient
    e. The left ventricular (LV) pressure and/or aortic pressure are not prognostic in PS

3. **All of the following angiographic features characterize dysplastic PS except:**
    a. Thickened pulmonary valve leaflets
    b. Hypoplastic pulmonary annulus
    c. Symmetric systolic doming of the pulmonary valve
    d. Absence of post-stenotic dilatation
    e. All of the above are true

4. **Which of the following statements regarding balloon valvuloplasty for PS is true?**
    a. The long-term results are characterized by recurrence in about one-third of patients
    b. The balloon size is based on the annular size: the smaller the size (predicted by age and body size), the better the results
    c. Pulmonary balloon valvuloplasty (PBV) is ineffective in patients with a dysplastic pulmonary valve
    d. Post-procedure pulmonary regurgitation is uncommon
    e. PBV is contraindicated in asymptomatic patients with moderate-to-severe PS

A 45-year-old woman has elevated PA and right ventricular (RV) systolic pressures with a continuous diastolic murmur across the right upper sternal border. There is no RV–PA systolic gradient. The RV and PA pressures (0–100 mmHg scale) are shown on Figure 5.2.

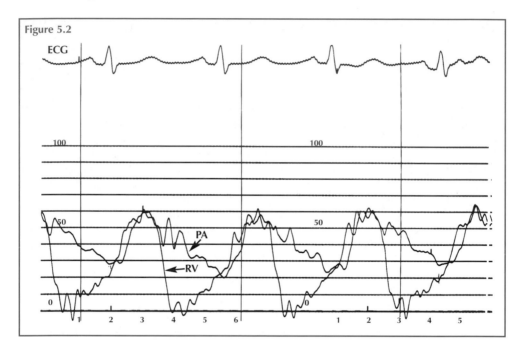

Figure 5.2

5. What is the most likely diagnosis based on Figure 5.2?
    a. PS
    b. VSD and PS
    c. Tetralogy of Fallot
    d. ASD
    e. Pulmonary valvular insufficiency

6. What is the most characteristic hemodynamic finding of this diagnosis?
    a. RV–PA gradient
    b. PA pulse pressure
    c. RV–PA end-diastolic pressures
    d. RV diastolic filling rate (slope)
    e. RV end-diastolic pressure (RVEDP)

Answers

1. **a** The diagnosis of PS with an intact ventricular septum is differentiated from that of an ASD or VSD by the absence of oxygen step-up at the atrial or ventricular level, respectively. The absence of cyanosis excludes typical tetralogy of Fallot. However, patients with PS may have cyanosis in the presence of patent foramen ovale or ASD.

   The differential diagnoses of moderate-to-severe PS with cyanosis include tetralogy of Fallot, VSD and PS. In patients without cyanosis, VSD associated with PS and left-to-right shunt would be a plausible diagnosis.

   Valvular PS with intact ventricular septum is a relatively common congenital malformation. It accounts for about 10% of all cardiac defects. Most of the patients are asymptomatic and will often be discovered during routine physical examination if a right-sided murmur is present. When present, symptoms vary from mild exertional dyspnea to frank congestive heart failure. Patients with moderate-to-severe PS can experience chest pain, syncope and even sudden cardiac death during exertion. Physical examination may reveal a palpable systolic thrill over the second and third spaces and a RV systolic impulse. Distinctive auscultatory features include a pulmonary ejection sound that decreases during inspiration. Systolic ejection-type murmur over the precordium is characteristic—its intensity is directly related to the severity of the stenosis. The duration and the peak of the murmur are longer and later, respectively, with increasing severity as the disease progresses.

   Cardiac catheterization is indicated to exclude associated abnormalities and demonstrate the severity and location of stenosis. Other associated hemodynamic findings include giant A-waves in the right atrial (RA) pressure tracing secondary to decreased RV compliance. The differential diagnoses of giant A-waves include junctional rhythm, tricuspid valve stenosis (slow Y-descent), PS or pulmonary hypertension (S₂ is single or closely split and loud, and the ejection systolic murmur is short, soft and localized to the left upper parasternal edge).

2. **c** In mild degrees of PS, the PA pressure is normal. In severe PS there is a marked reduction of the mean PA pressure and obliteration of the usual pulsatile configuration of the pressure tracing.

   Gorlin's formula can be used only with isolated stenosis of the aortic and mitral valves. In the presence of associated infundibular stenosis, calculation of the valve area using this formula is not valid. The formula measures flow across an orifice rather than across an elongated tube or across more than one site of obstruction.

   The stroke volume does not increase in patients with severe obstruction but remains normal or slightly decreased. In the study of congenital heart disease, heart rate is the most important correlate of peak systolic pressure gradient across the pulmonary valve. When the pressure gradient is adjusted for the heart rate (i.e. systolic ejection period), adding cardiac output to the calculation does not improve the correlation with the gradient.

The classification of PS into mild, moderate and severe is based on the correlations between clinical and hemodynamic observations. When the resting RV pressure is <50 mmHg, the stenosis is characterized as mild. In moderate PS, the pressures in the RV and LV are equal. RV systolic pressure is higher than systemic pressure in patients with severe PS.

3. c The valves are not fused in dysplastic PS, but because they are thickened they are relatively immobile. The main pulmonary trunk is hypoplastic, further limiting the mobility of the valve. Other characteristic features include asymmetric valve doming, no systolic 'jet' and no post-stenotic dilatation.

The stenotic pulmonary valve is dome-shaped and projects toward the PA. It is formed by fusion of the leaflets. In 10–15% of cases, a dysplastic valve is obstructing outflow. The dysplastic valve is exceptionally thick and the annulus is narrow. The leaflets are not fused and hence there is no post-stenotic dilatation. The RV, especially the infundibular region, is hypertrophied in patients with PS. Post-stenotic dilatation of the pulmonary trunk is also present, which is not seen in patients with dysplastic valves.

Two-dimensional echocardiography can differentiate valvular, sub- and supra-valvular stenosis and dysplastic valves.

4. c The results of PBV for isolated PS are excellent. If the pulmonary valve annulus is near normal size (>75% of the size predicted for age and body surface area), valvuloplasty will be highly effective. However, it is ineffective in a dysplastic pulmonary valve. PBV is indicated in patients with moderate and severe PS.

PBV is the treatment of choice for PS. The size of the balloon should be at least 10–20% larger than the pulmonary valve annulus. If the annulus is more than 20 mm in diameter, it may be necessary to use two balloons simultaneously.

Surgical valvotomy is an excellent alternative to PBV. Most surgical valvotomies are done under direct vision, approaching the valve through an incision in the pulmonary trunk. In the post-operative period, a systolic gradient across the RV outflow tract (RVOT) may persist for a few hours. Rarely, fatal RV failure ensues secondary to hypercontraction of the infundibular area (suicidal RV). Propranolol relieves hypercontractile RV outflow obstruction but not residual valvular obstruction. In the case of a dysplastic pulmonary valve, removing the thickened valve tissue and enlarging the annulus and proximal PA by inserting a patch may relieve outflow obstruction.

5. e

6. d The hemodynamics of pulmonary insufficiency correspond to those seen for acute aortic insufficiency, where RVEDP increases (25 mmHg) and nearly equals that of PA diastolic pressure at the onset of RV contraction. The elevated PA diastolic pressure alone does not indicate pulmonary insufficiency; it should be accompanied by marked distortion of diastolic RV pressure and continued filling of the RV.

Chapter 6
Hypertrophic Cardiomyopathy

A young man undergoes cardiac catheterization to evaluate increasing dyspnea on exertion and a systolic ejection murmur. Simultaneous high fidelity recordings from the left atrium (LA), aortic root (AoR), left ventricular outflow tract (LVOT) and mid left ventricle (LV) are displayed (Figure 6.1).

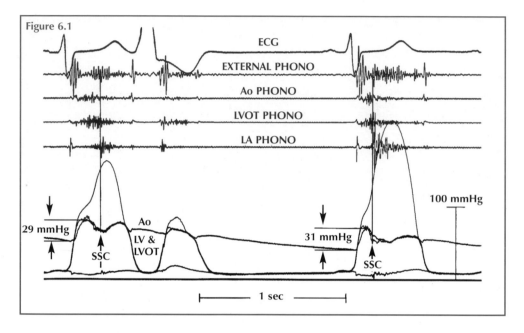

Figure 6.1

1. Which of the following are demonstrated by the hemodynamic changes on tracing Figure 6.1?
   a. Aortic stenosis (AS)
   b. Hypertrophic cardiomyopathy (HCM)
   c. Aortic regurgitation
   d. Mitral regurgitation (MR)
   e. Supra-Ao valvular stenosis

2. Which of the following maneuvers may increase an LV–Ao systolic gradient in patients with HCM?
   a. Amyl nitrite inhalation
   b. Squatting
   c. Phenylephrine infusion
   d. Passive leg raising
   e. Handgrip

A 45-year-old man was found to have a harsh systolic murmur. He reports the recent onset of exertional chest discomfort, and a syncopal episode one year ago. At cardiac catheterization, the following hemodynamic tracing was recorded (Figure 6.2).

Figure 6.2

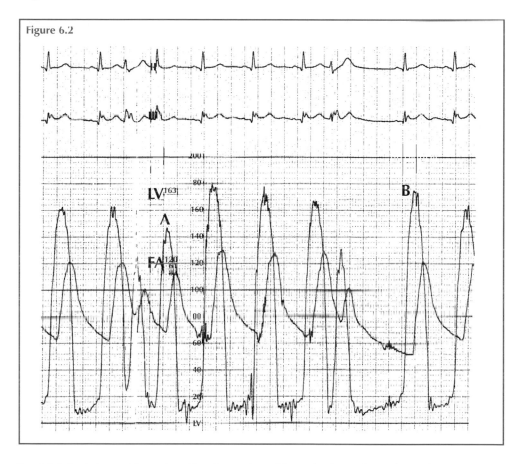

3. Which statement best describes beats A and B on the hemodynamic tracing (Figure 6.2)?
   a. The post-extrasystolic beat labeled 'A' demonstrates a decrease in Ao pulse pressure consistent with the Brockenbrough effect
   b. The post-extrasystolic beat labeled 'B' demonstrates an increase in the LV outflow gradient seen only in HCM
   c. The post-extrasystolic beat labeled 'B' is most consistent with a fixed outflow obstruction
   d. The post-extrasystolic beat labeled 'B' demonstrates the effects of a non-compensatory pause on the pressure gradient
   e. The difference in the post-extrasystolic gradient in the beats labeled 'A' and 'B' is best explained by a relative increase in augmented contractility in 'B'

4. Regarding the hemodynamic tracing (Figure 6.3), all of the following statements are true except:
   a. The carotid pulse may be diminished (in volume) and delayed compared to the apical impulse
   b. In supra-valvular stenosis, the coronary arteries may be exposed to supra-physiologic pressures
   c. The observed hemodynamic tracing may be seen in patients with a discrete sub-Ao membrane
   d. The observed hemodynamic tracing may be seen in patients with bicuspid Ao valve stenosis
   e. Wolff-Parkinson-White syndrome is a known associated finding

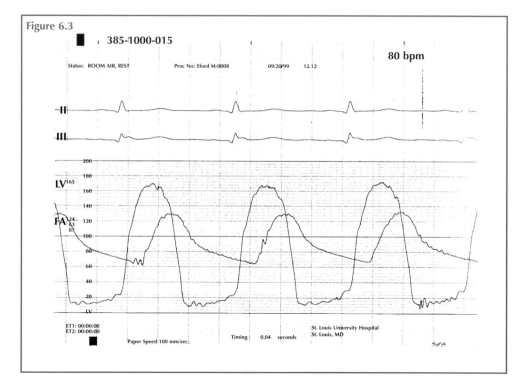

Figure 6.3

5. Which of the following physical findings is least likely to be observed in the patient (Figure 6.3)?
   a. Ao insufficiency
   b. MR
   c. Ejection click
   d. Elfin facies
   e. Systolic murmur at the supra-sternal notch

A 32-year-old male has had a systolic murmur since childhood. Echocardiography indicates mild concentric LV hypertrophy with both septal and posterior wall thickness of 1.2 cm without resting or provokable intra-cavitary gradient. His LV–Ao tracing is shown in Figure 6.4.

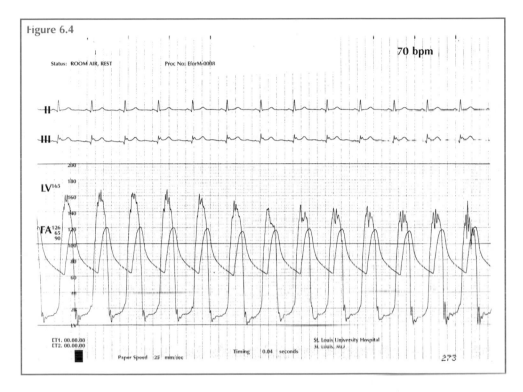

Figure 6.4

6. From the hemodynamic tracing in Figure 6.4, which of the following is most likely to be present on physical exam?
   a. The carotid pulse is diminished and late
   b. The carotid pulse is hyperkinetic
   c. The associated systolic murmur increases with the Valsalva maneuver
   d. The associated diastolic murmur decreases with sustained handgrip
   e. An ejection click is commonly observed

7. Which of the following echocardiographic findings are associated with the diagnosis in Figure 6.4?
   a. Bicuspid Ao valve
   b. Continuous wave Doppler of the LVOT demonstrating a dagger-shaped trace (peak gradient in late systole)
   c. Persistent systolic and diastolic echo densities seen in the LVOT
   d. Eccentric LV hypertrophy
   e. Systolic anterior motion of the mitral valve leaflets

An asymptomatic 18-year-old male college student who participates in collegiate sports comes for a routine physical examination. A III/VI systolic ejection murmur is heard at the lower left sternal border. The electrocardiogram (ECG) shows LV hypertrophy. Echocardiographic study reveals a LV septal wall thickness of 20 mm. LV and Ao hemodynamic tracings are obtained at catheterization.

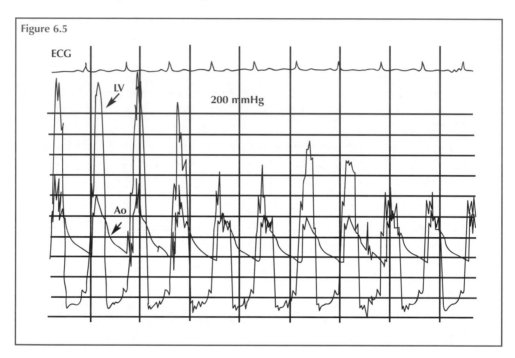

Figure 6.5

8. Based on the hemodynamic tracing (Figure 6.5), what is the most likely diagnosis?
   a. Mitral stenosis (MS)
   b. AS
   c. HCM
   d. Supra-valvular Stenosis
   e. Pulmonary stenosis

9. Which of the following is the most diagnostic finding?
   a. LV–Ao pressure gradient
   b. Wide pulse pressure
   c. Delayed Ao pressure upstroke
   d. Post-premature ventricular contraction (PVC) reduction of LV–Ao gradient
   e. Reduction of LV–Ao gradient on pullback from LV apex to a sub-valvular position.

10. Which of the following findings may be seen with valvular AS but not HCM?
    a. 'Spike and dome' configuration of Ao pressure
    b. Large A-wave on LV tracing
    c. Widened pulse pressure
    d. Exaggerated LV–Ao gradient with isometric handgrip
    e. Delayed upstroke of Ao pressure

11. Maneuvers are often performed to further substantiate the diagnosis. In the tracing in Figure 6.6, what is the diagnostic maneuver associated with HCM?
    a. Phenylephrine infusion
    b. Isometric handgrip
    c. Beta-receptor blockade
    d. Squatting
    e. PVCs

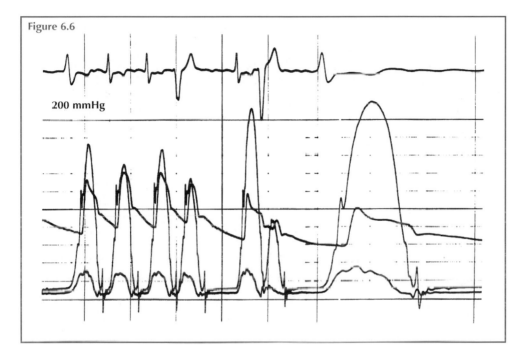

Figure 6.6

200 mmHg

12. What additional findings are present in Figure 6.6 that are associated with HCM?
    a. Delayed upstroke of Ao pressure
    b. 'Spike and dome' of Ao pressure
    c. Narrow dicrotic notch
    d. Increased left ventricular end-diastolic pressure (LVEDP)
    e. Widened pulse pressure when in normal sinus rhythm

Catheter-based therapy has been instituted for the 18-year-old patient with HCM. Figure 6.7 shows hemodynamics after treatment.

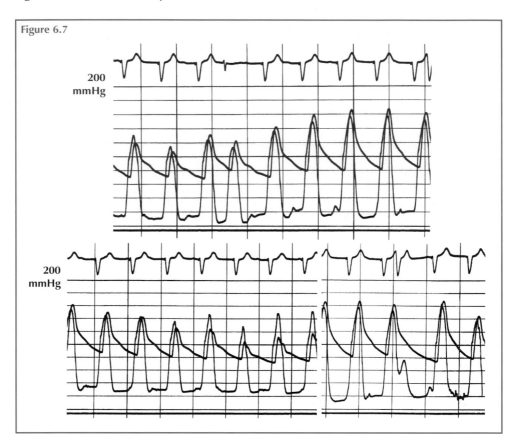

Figure 6.7

200 mmHg

200 mmHg

13. Which of the following therapies was employed?
    a. Digitalis
    b. Isoproterenol
    c. Amyl nitrate
    d. Alcohol
    e. Tegretol

14. Based on the hemodynamic tracing in Figure 6.7, all of the following indicate procedural success, except :
    a. Valsalva provokable LV–Ao gradient <30 mmHg
    b. Absence of Brockenbrough-Braunwald-Morrow sign
    c. High-grade heart block
    d. Resting LV–Ao gradient <10 mmHg
    e. Post-PVC gradient <30 mmHg

Answers

1. **b** HCM is distinctive in that invasive hemodynamic recordings often reveal a dynamic pressure gradient in the sub-Ao area of the LVOT. A large systolic gradient between the LV and the Ao is seen on the first and third beats. Following a premature ventricular beat (second beat) in HCM patients, the Ao pulse pressure is unchanged and the systolic pressure gradient is increased. Both AS and HCM can produce an increased systolic gradient following a PVC. However, in HCM the peripheral pulse pressure is reduced or at least fails to increase as expected (Brockenbrough-Braunwald-Morrow sign) due to post-PVC inotropic potentiation leading to an increased degree of outflow obstruction. The resulting increased obstruction to LV outflow is often associated with a decreased Ao pressure pulse. A dynamic obstruction to outflow is not often present in AS, where both the LV and Ao pressures usually increase post-PVC. Gentle advancement of the pigtail catheter can be used to induce a PVC. Inotropic stimulation with beta-agonists (such as dobutamine or isoproterenol) may provoke an LV outflow gradient in suspected HCM cases.

   In cases of Ao and supra-Ao valvular stenoses, the pulse pressure is increased following a PVC, and the LV–Ao pressure gradient remains relatively constant. Dilated cardiomyopathy will not produce a systolic gradient (unless AS is present), although LV systolic function may be augmented post PVC on imaging studies. An example of the post PVC augmentation in AS is shown on Figure 6.8. Note the increased Ao pulse pressure, systolic gradient and associated ejection murmur.

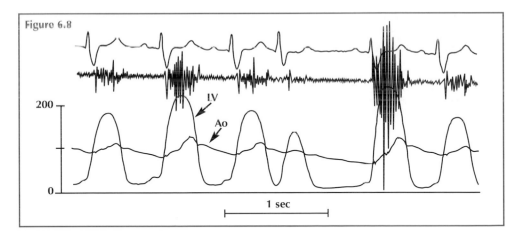

Figure 6.8

200

0

1 sec

LV

Ao

2. **a** Hemodynamic maneuvers can differentiate LV–Ao systolic gradients or outflow murmurs caused by valvular, supra-valvular, sub-valvular or intraventricular pathology.

   Maneuvers or drugs that decrease LV preload will exaggerate the dynamic systolic gradient. Amyl nitrate administered by inhalation has a transient hemodynamic effect causing both arterial and venodilation. The resulting decrease in both preload (venous return) and afterload is associated with an increased sub-valvular obstruction to flow. Mitral regurgitation may also be exaggerated as a result of an increased anterior mitral valve leaflet displacement secondary to the Venturi effect associated with an accelerated flow velocity through the region of obstruction.

Phenylephrine (an arterial vasoconstrictor that increases afterload) reduces the systolic pressure gradient by increasing Ao diastolic pressure. Isometric handgrip similarly produces an increased afterload. Both passive leg elevation and the Müller maneuver (forced and sustained inspiration against a closed glottis) increase preload. In accordance with the Frank-Starling principle, an increased preload requires a lessened systolic contractile force to maintain cardiac output. The sub-valvular dynamic obstruction is thereby decreased. Squatting produces both increased preload and increased afterload.

3. c   The post-extrasystolic (post-PVC) beat labeled 'B' shows an increase in both the LV–Ao gradient and the Ao pulse pressure, consistent with a fixed obstruction to LV outflow. These findings are explained by an increase in LV volume due to prolonged and compensatory diastolic filling following the PVC, and by an increase in LV contractility following the extrasystolic beat. This post-extrasystolic potentiation of contractile force can be explained by the force-frequency relation often referred to as the 'Bowditch staircase phenomenon' or 'Treppe' (steps in German) effect. The increased force of contraction is similar in mechanism to that seen with increasing heart rates. An increased gradient and Ao pulse pressure are seen in fixed sub-valvular, valvular or supra-valvular stenosis. The Brockenbrough effect, characteristic of HCM, describes a decrease in Ao pulse pressure despite an increase in LV contractility resulting from a dynamic outflow tract obstruction (the increase in post-extrasystolic contractility far outweighs the mitigating effect of the increased diastolic filling period).

Answer 'b' is incorrect, as a post-PVC increase in the outflow pressure gradient is seen in both fixed and dynamic obstructions due to increased volumetric LV filling. However, in this case the Ao pulse pressure increases, which is not suggestive of HCM.

Answer 'a' is incorrect, as the beat labeled 'A' follows an interpolated extrasystolic beat. The shortened diastolic period leads to a decrease in LV filling, and therefore a decrease in both the gradient and the Ao pulse pressure.

Answer 'd' is incorrect, as the post-PVC beat labeled 'B' follows a compensatory pause, wherein the interval surrounding the PVC is twice the basic cycle length. The only significance of this difference is the prolonged filling period compared to a non-compensatory pause or interpolated PVC.

Answer 'e' is incorrect, as the main difference between beats 'A' and 'B' is the markedly shortened diastolic filling period for beat 'A'. An increase in contractility is expected in both beats 'A' and 'B'.

4. e   In contrast to HCM, in all fixed LV–Ao obstructions the upstroke of the Ao pressure trace is delayed into late systole (the angle of the Ao pressure upslope is reduced). This tracing is representative of a fixed outflow tract obstruction, such as valvular AS, and either supra-valvular or sub-valvular obstructions to flow. In the case of supra-valvular obstruction, the most common site is the sinotubular junction above the coronary ostia, exposing the coronary arteries to the increased LV pressures rather than the limited Ao pressures measured peripherally, beyond the level of obstruction to flow.

Wolff-Parkinson-White syndrome is associated with HCM, but not other forms of fixed LV–Ao obstruction.

In contrast to fixed Ao obstruction, the Ao waveform in HCM characteristically demonstrates a rapid early upstroke, with the initial upstroke of the Ao trace mirroring that of the LV upstroke, and the LV systolic waveform appearing 'dagger-like' (see Figures 6.1 and 6.9). The Ao waveform often is described as a 'spike and dome' pattern. In hypertrophic (obstructive) cardiomyopathy (HCM), the interventricular septum is asymmetrically hypertrophied to a greater extent than the LV free wall. Both Doppler echocardiography and catheterization will reveal an intra-cavitary gradient. Continuous wave LV outflow Doppler interrogations often have a characteristic 'dagger' shape similar to LV pressures recorded directly in the catheterization laboratory.

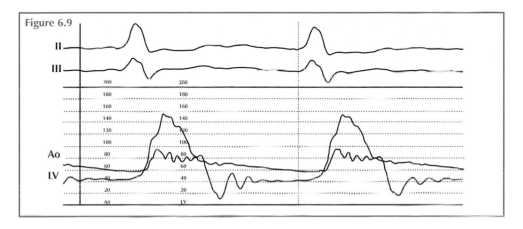

Figure 6.9

5. **b** Aortic valve regurgitation (AR) is commonly observed in sub Ao obstructions (secondary to leaflet trauma from the acceleration and turbulence of flow through the sub-Ao membrane) as well as valvular AS. An ejection click may be appreciated in either acquired Ao or congenital bicuspid Ao valve stenosis, though not in sub-AS patients.

Elfin facies is a characteristic of Williams-Beuren syndrome, which is found in 30% of patients with supravalvular fixed AS. Other findings of this syndrome include mental retardation, infantile hypercalcemia, peripheral pulmonary or systemic artery stenosis, and dental anomalies. In supra-valvular AS, differential peripheral pressures may occur (right arm greater than left arm, and greater than the femoral pressure), and the murmur is loudly transmitted to the neck and suprasternal notch.

Mitral regurgitation is appreciated in many patients with HCM, but is unusual in other forms of fixed obstruction to LV outflow. As long as rheumatic valvular heart disease is excluded as an etiologic explanation for multi-valvular disease, answer 'b' is the least likely associated finding.

6. **a** Since HCM is excluded by echocardiography, and pullback of the end-hole-only catheter within the LV demonstrates that the LV–Ao gradient is below the Ao valve, sub-Ao obstruction is the diagnosis. This finding is confirmed by the absence of a pressure gradient while the catheter tip remains within the LV. In fixed sub AS, many of the physical findings are the same as with valvular AS. Therefore, the carotid pulse may be diminished in volume and delayed (*parvus et tardus*).

In HCM, the carotid pulse is hyperkinetic (and may be bisferiens). A mid-cavitary gradient may also be observed with HCM, though the Ao pulse contour of Figure 6.4 is not consistent with this diagnosis. The strain phase (phase II) of the Valsalva maneuver causes a decreased venous return, thereby accentuating the systolic murmur of HCM but decreasing murmurs from fixed outflow obstructions (see Figure 6.9).
Sustained handgrip, or any other maneuver that increases systemic vascular resistance, exacerbates a diastolic Ao regurgitation murmur, which is frequently present in cases of sub-valvular obstruction.

An ejection click is rarely heard in fixed sub-valvular stenosis, but it is common in congenital bicuspid AS, although it may disappear as the patient ages with progressive thickening of the valve leaflets.

7. c Discrete membranes or myocardial ridges are often seen in cases of sub-Ao obstruction to LV outflow suggested by persistent echo densities parallel to the Ao valve in the outflow tract. Doppler echocardiography will often reveal the fixed intra-cavitary gradient.

Echocardiography has supplanted cardiac catheterization for establishing a definitive diagnosis of obstructions to LV outflow. Sub-aortic stenosis causes a fixed obstruction to LV outflow frequently due to a discrete membrane, thickened muscular ridge or fibromuscular tunnel. Mild to moderate AR is common due to valve leaflet trauma induced by acceleration and turbulence of the LV systolic jet through the narrowed outflow tract. During cardiac catheterization, the Ao waveforms of fixed outflow obstruction (recorded distal to the site of obstruction) are similar and demonstrate a delayed slope and peaking of the systolic pressure. Careful pullback of the LV catheter will reveal the site of intra-cavitary obstruction. Left ventriculography may demonstrate either a narrowing of the LVOT or a discrete membrane.

Congenital bicuspid Ao valves are a common cause of Ao valvular stenosis in young patients. Continuous wave Doppler of the LVOT demonstrating a dagger-shaped trace peaking late in systole is characteristic of HCM. The Venturi effect of turbulence in the LVOT (pulling the anterior mitral valve leaflet into the LVOT, interrupting leaflet coaptation) is a commonly accepted explanation for mitral regurgitation seen with HCM. Eccentric LV hypertrophy is not associated with pressure-overload states such as fixed obstructions to LV outflow, but is commonly seen with volume-overload states such as either severe Ao or mitral insufficiency.

8. c Catheter pullback (from left to right side of tracing) demonstrates LV pressure reduction with LV systolic pressure equal to Ao pressure once the sub-valvular obstruction in the ventricular chamber is passed.

9. e Both HCM and other forms of AS have LV–Ao gradients. Only the fixed forms of AS are associated with delayed Ao pressure upstroke. The post-extrasystolic LV–Ao pressure gradient is either preserved or increased in both fixed stenosis or HCM.

A widened pulse pressure may be seen in sub-valvular stenosis if significant Ao regurgitation is also present.

10. e HCM has an initial rapid rise in Ao pressure associated with vigorous LV ejection, producing a spike followed by dome waveform. This spike and dome may be palpable as a bisferiens pulse. A widened pulse pressure is associated with Ao insufficiency. Handgrip increases afterload and decreases the LV–Ao gradient in both conditions. The Ao upstroke is delayed in (fixed) Ao valve stenosis.

11. e A PVC potentiates the post-extrasystolic gradient and reduces the pulse pressure. The reduction of the pulse pressure of the following beat is characteristic of HCM. The other maneuvers will reduce the LV–Ao gradients in HCM.

12. b The rapid LV ejection with abrupt outflow obstruction causes a peak, or 'spike', and delayed remaining ejection phase, the 'dome'. The remaining findings are not characteristic, and not present on the tracing. HCM is not associated with Ao regurgitation and does not cause a widened pulse pressure.

13. d Focal myonecrosis of a bulging septal wall segment can be successfully induced by instillation of denatured alcohol selectively into the first and/or second septal branches. This specialized technique, called percutaneous transluminal septal myocardial ablation (PTSMA), results in improved symptoms and a reduction in the dynamic LV–Ao gradient. Digitalis and isoproterenol both accentuate myocardial contractility, exaggerating the degree of obstruction. Amyl nitrate inhalation reduces both preload and afterload, exaggerating the degree of (dynamic) obstruction. Other modalities that may be employed to reduce the LV–Ao gradient in HCM include permanent pacing (note widened QRS on this tracing, although no P-wave is visible and dual-chamber devices are preferable), beta-blockade administration (decreases contractility), or alpha-adrenoreceptor stimulation (phenylephrine; increases afterload).

14. c All of the hemodynamic changes noted are associated with a successful procedure. Complete heart block may occur in 5–20% of patients treated with PTSMA, and is considered a complication of the procedure.

Chapter 7
Diastolic Dysfunction

A 50-year-old male with fatigue, atypical chest pain and a systolic murmur was referred for cardiac catheterization. Initial hemodynamic pressures are recorded on Figure 7.1, panel A. Within a few minutes of inserting the pigtail catheter, recordings on panel B were obtained.

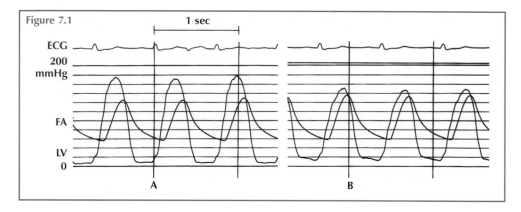

1. The hemodynamic changes between panels A and B are most likely due to which of the following?
   a. Severe aortic stenosis
   b. Acute aortic regurgitation
   c. Severe combined aortic stenosis and regurgitation
   d. Carabello's sign
   e. Malposition of the pigtail catheter

Simultaneous left ventricular (LV) and pulmonary capillary wedge (PCW) hemodynamic recordings (Figure 7.2) were obtained from a 59-year-old woman 10 days after an inferior myocardial infarction.

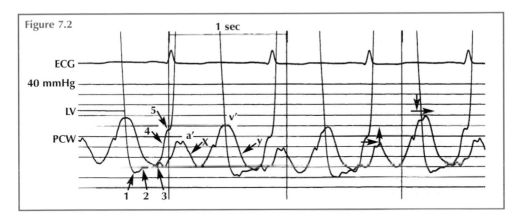

Figure 7.2

2. The most appropriate location on the LV waveform to determine LV end-diastolic pressure (LVEDP) is?
   a. 1
   b. 2
   c. 3
   d. 4
   e. 5

3. Which of the following statements is true for the hemodynamic evaluation of PCW pressures?
   a. The discrepancy between LVED and PCW pressures is often ≥5 mmHg
   b. The timing delay of PCW pressure relative to left atrial (LA) pressure is usually ≤40 msec
   c. PCW pressures are easily obtained in patients with tricuspid regurgitation, pulmonary hypertension or a dilated right ventricle (RV)
   d. PCW pressure is not a reliable indicator of LA and LVED pressures in most patients
   e. Oxygen saturation obtained in the wedge position nearing that of aortic blood can be used to confirm appropriate PCW pressure waveforms and wedge position

A 72-year-old woman with severe three-vessel coronary artery disease and hypertension presents with unstable angina. Hemodynamic tracings of her LV pressure before and after administration of nitroglycerin (NTG) are shown on Figure 7.3.

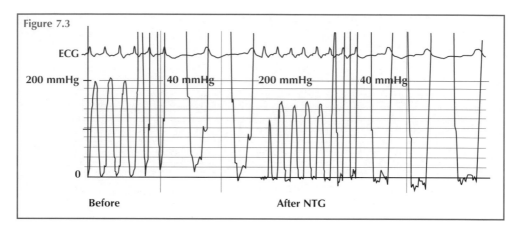

Figure 7.3

4. **What is the LVEDP before NTG administration in Figure 7.3?**
    a. 10 mmHg
    b. 20 mmHg
    c. 30 mmHg
    d. 40 mmHg
    e. LVEDP cannot be determined due to catheter artifact

5. **Which of the following statements is true regarding the effects of NTG administration in the patient described in Figure 7.3?**
    a. LV preload is increased
    b. LV systolic pressure remains unchanged
    c. Both LV systolic and diastolic volumes increase
    d. The LV pressure-volume relationship is shifted leftwards
    e. Myocardial oxygen demand is increased after receiving NTG

6. **In which tracing is the LV diastolic waveform associated with impaired ventricular relaxation?**
    a. Figure 7.4 top (scale 0–40 mmHg)
    b. Figure 7.5 (scale 0–40 mmHg)
    c. Figure 7.6 (scale 0–40 mmHg)
    d. Figure 7.7 (scale 0–40 mmHg)

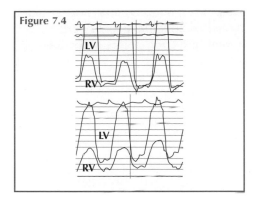

Figure 7.4

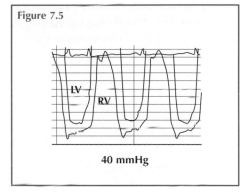

Figure 7.5

40 mmHg

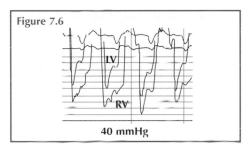

Figure 7.6

40 mmHg

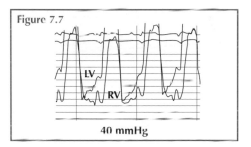

Figure 7.7

40 mmHg

7. In Figure 7.6, why is the RV pressure upstroke delayed relative to the LV pressure wave?
   a. Constrictive pericarditis
   b. LV pre-excitation
   c. LV failure
   d. Pacemaker rhythm
   e. Right bundle branch block

8. In Figure 7.7, examination of the RV and LV diastolic pressures indicates which of the following:
   a. LV compliance is high
   b. RV compliance is low
   c. LV compliance is low
   d. RV shows constrictive physiology
   e. LV shows constrictive physiology

The LV pressure was recorded continuously (Figures 7.8 and 7.9) in a 43-year-old woman with exertional chest pain and multiple risk factors for coronary artery disease. The tracings demonstrate several different inflection points of the A-wave and LVEDP.

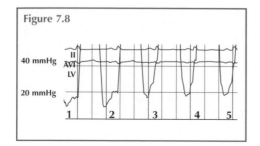

Figure 7.8

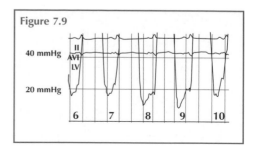

Figure 7.9

9. Based on Figures 7.8 and 7.9, what is the true LVEDP?
   a. 5 mmHg
   b. 10 mmHg
   c. 20 mmHg
   d. 30 mmHg
   e. 40 mmHg

10. Why is the LVEDP on Figures 7.8 and 7.9 changing?
    a. Respiratory variation
    b. Catheter artifact
    c. Impaired LV relaxation
    d. Tamponade
    e. Constriction

A 42-year-old man with hypertension and atypical chest pain syndrome undergoes catheterization with LV pressure measurements (Figure 7.10).

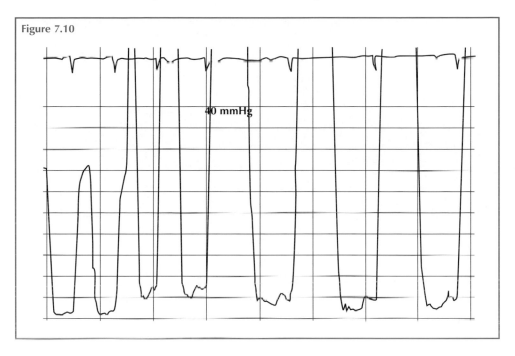

Figure 7.10

40 mmHg

11. The pressure waveforms shown in Figure 7.10 suggest which of the following findings?
   a. Constriction
   b. Tamponade
   c. Congestive heart failure
   d. Normal LV function
   e. Diastolic dysfunction

Answers

1. e On panel B, one or more of the side holes of the pigtail catheter has moved into the aorta, demonstrated by the higher initial LV diastolic pressure and progressive decline (downsloping) of LV pressure across diastole. This catheter artifact becomes more recognizable as more side holes open within the aorta, resulting in the initial LV diastolic pressure becoming even more elevated to a level approaching that of aortic diastolic pressure. Note the identical aortic pressure between tracings.

Carabello's sign is an increase of ≥5 mmHg in peripheral artery pressure when the LV catheter is withdrawn across a severely stenotic aortic valve, reflecting the obstruction to flow (and pressure) from the catheter itself. Aortic regurgitation does not influence the Ao root–LV pressures as shown here.

2. e LVEDP is obtained after atrial contraction at the end of the A-wave. LVEDP is measured after the A-wave corresponding to the onset of the electrocardiographic 'R' wave.

3. e Normally, PCW pressure approximates both LA and LVED pressures, assuming the absence of mitral stenosis. In certain disease states that are associated with an elevated pulmonary vascular resistance (hypoxemia, pulmonary embolism and pulmonary hypertension), and occasionally after mitral valve surgery, the PCW may not accurately reflect LA pressure. Furthermore, PCW pressure may not accurately reflect LVEDP in the setting of diastolic dysfunction. It can be difficult to obtain a true PCW pressure recording in some patients with pulmonary hypertension due to waveform contamination or difficulty in wedging the balloon properly. Tricuspid regurgitation or a dilated RV both impede balloon-catheter rotation without fluoroscopic guidance. The timing delay of PCW pressure relative to LA pressure is usually 40–120 msec. An oxygen saturation nearing that of systemic arterial saturation confirms correct wedge position.

4. b The LVEDP at the R-wave is 18–22 mmHg (20 mmHg average). An LVEDP of >30 mmHg has been associated with the development of both accelerated angina and acute congestive heart failure after left ventriculography. LVEDP elevation nearing 40 mmHg is a sign of impending pulmonary edema and is usually an indication for urgent treatment with aggressive preload and afterload reduction and/or intra-aortic balloon counterpulsation.

5. d Nitrates rapidly increase venous capacitance, thereby reducing venous return. The decreased venous return to the right heart is reflected through the pulmonary circuit and reducing LV filling volumes and pressures. A downward and leftward shift in the LV pressure-volume curve occurs. Myocardial oxygen demand is reduced because of a reduced mechanical wall stress on the myocardium. Note the decreased systolic and LVED pressures after NTG.

6. b Diastolic dysfunction is defined as the inability of the LV to relax normally, impairing volumetric filling. This condition results in elevated end-diastolic pressures and decreased end-diastolic volumes, ultimately leading to decreased forward stroke volume and symptoms of low cardiac output or pulmonary congestion. Diastole is frequently divided into four phases: isovolumic relaxation, early filling, diastasis and atrial systole. Myocardial compliance and the rate at which the ventricles relax affect each phase of diastole.

Normally, active myocardial relaxation begins before aortic valve closure and is usually complete by the middle of diastole. Therefore, it does not influence either diastasis or active filling from atrial systole. Cardiomyopathies, due to ischemia or hypertrophy, delay both the active and passive phases of ventricular relaxation. With disease progression, there is a greater relative atrial contribution to ventricular filling in an attempt to maintain ventricular volume. Thus larger A-waves are commonly seen in LV pressure tracings.

LA pressure is an important determinant of early diastolic filling. In severe situations, LA pressures increase in an attempt to restore early diastolic filling volumes to normal at the expense of elevated atrial and ventricular filling pressures.

Diastolic dysfunction, a restrictive form of ventricular filling, is characterized by a prolonged isovolumic relaxation time (IVRT). Although no filling occurs during IVRT, this process greatly influences ventricular filling after the mitral valve opens. With diastolic dysfunction, the lowest recorded LV diastolic pressures may not occur until the middle of diastole. The time constant of ventricular relaxation [τ (tau)] is a precise measurement of the rate of decrease of ventricular pressure during isovolumic relaxation and can be determined invasively during catheterization from the slope of the LV pressure wave during isovolumetric relaxation. An increase in τ directly correlates with abnormal ventricular relaxation and the degree of diastolic dysfunction.

Additionally, passive stiffness of the myocardium is increased by fibrosis resulting from recurrent ischemia, infarction or an infiltrating process. Myocyte hypertrophy, induced by poorly controlled hypertension or valvular heart disease, also increases stiffness. The last phase of diastole, atrial contraction, contributes 15–25% of the ventricular diastolic volume, but in certain disease states this contribution can be as high as 40%. The atrial contribution to ventricular filling will be even greater in patients with diminished early relaxation. The ventricular diastolic pressure-volume relationship may be abnormal because of changes in active relaxation, passive compliance properties or both. The final result is impaired ventricular filling with typical LV diastolic waveform and inappropriately elevated LA and pulmonary venous pressures.

Restrictive cardiomyopathies (sarcoidosis, hemochromatosis and amyloidosis) may cause increased passive chamber stiffness from deposition of the implicated substance in the myocardium or interstitial space, and have characteristic RV-LV filling curves. Aging, independent of other disease processes, may prolong LV relaxation.

Diastolic dysfunction may cause symptoms of both dyspnea and fatigue, secondary to an inadequate increase in cardiac output, despite normal systolic function. If systolic function is also abnormal, these symptoms may be exaggerated.

Although the LVEDP in Figure 7.5 is only 16 mmHg, there is an impaired LV diastolic pressure waveform of abnormal relaxation. The LV diastolic tracing does not reach its minimum nadir until mid-diastole, suggesting an impairment in isovolumic relaxation.

In Figure 7.4 (top) the LVEDP is normal at 8–10 mmHg. The RV pressure is also normal. The electrocardiographic junctional rhythm does not demonstrate P-waves, thus explaining the absence of the A-wave on the LVEDP. This tracing does not demonstrate any significant diastolic functional pathology with the exception of a junctional rhythm and relatively low-normal filling pressures.

Figure 7.4 (bottom) shows biventricular failure with elevation of minimal and end-diastolic pressures, but normal (early) isovolumic relaxation.

Figures 7.6 and 7.7 also show increased LVEDP with rapid filling across diastole, but normal (early) isovolumic relaxation.

7. e Abnormalities of cardiac conduction produce marked distortions in the timing relationship between the ejection onset of LV and RV pressures. In Figure 7.6, the LVEDP is 32 mmHg and the RVEDP is 22 mmHg. The alignment of ventricular pressures provides a clue to conduction abnormalities, if not already evident from the electrocardiographic tracings. In this case, the delayed RV pressure upstroke (relative to the LV) suggests RV conduction system delay.

8. c Although the patient also has a right bundle branch block (Figure 7.7) and an elevated LVEDP of 28 mmHg, gradual upslope of the waveform reflects the compliance of the LV. The rapid LV upslope greatly exceeds that of the RV upslope; the compliance of the LV (estimated from the slope of the diastolic filling pressure) can be compared to the rather slow filling rate (higher compliance) of the RV. Conditions of concentric hypertrophy, restrictive or infiltrative cardiomyopathy, or other diseases of the ventricular myocardium produce a stiffer LV wall, thus altering the pressure-volume curve and elevating the LVEDP.

The tracing does not demonstrate the characteristic 'dip and plateau' seen in constrictive (pericarditis) physiology, where most LV filling occurs very early. The rapid (early) diastolic filling is abruptly halted when the intracardiac volume reaches the peak plateau (or crest) pressure, representing the limitation against further volume expansion set by the non-compliant pericardium.

9. c The LVEDP immediately precedes isometric ventricular contraction in the LV pressure pulse. This point, also known as the Z-point, is situated on the downslope of the LV A-wave and marks the crossing over of the LA and LV pressures. The LVEDP is normally <12 mmHg. Impairment of myocardial contractility or changes in LV volume alter the diastolic pressure-volume relationship and shift the end-diastolic pressure point upward.

10. b A multiple-holed catheter (pigtail) may bridge the aortic valve and cause the LV to have an artifactually higher diastolic pressure. In this tracing, minor differences in positioning over the respiratory cycle of the pigtail catheter, with one or two of the side holes across the aortic valve, are the cause of the abnormally aligned LVEDP. Examining the diastolic pressure waveform and identifying the lowest LV pressure at the initiation of diastole can detect this artifact. The initial downstroke of LV pressure is delayed further, suggesting aortic pressure contamination by side-holes of the catheter having moved out of the LV. Catheter stability is needed for a reliable pressure wave in the interpretation of the LVEDP.

11. e The LV wave form demonstrates continuing decline of pressure over the mid-diastolic period, with the pressure nadir occurring more than halfway through the diastolic period. This is characteristic of diastolic dysfunction and impaired myocardial relaxation. This patient was found to have severe LV hypertrophy by echocardiography. Constriction and tamponade are not likely, given the low LV diastolic pressures shown. Congestive heart failure is a clinical diagnosis, and cannot be definitively identified using LV pressure measurements in isolation. LVEDP is usually, but not always, elevated in CHF patients, depending on volume status at the time of invasive monitoring.

Chapter 8

Tamponade

A 52-year-old man with hepatitis B and AIDS presented to the emergency department with a 1-week history of progressive dyspnea, chills, night sweats and increased abdominal girth. On examination, his respiratory rate was 24/minute. He had jugular venous pulsations at the angle of the jaw and bilateral submandibular lymphadenopathy. The lungs were clear. The heart sounds were distant. The electrocardiogram (ECG) revealed sinus tachycardia and low voltage QRS. The admission chest radiograph showed cardiomegaly and a mediastinal mass.

Computerized tomography of the chest revealed bilateral axillary, mediastinal, deep pelvic and inguinal adenopathy, a large pericardial effusion, bilateral pleural effusions and ascites. The arterial pressure is shown on Figure 8.1.

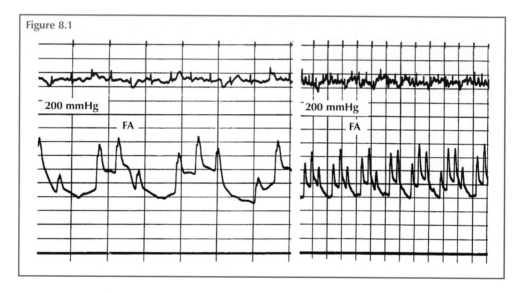

Figure 8.1

1. This patient's arterial pressure (Figure 8.1) shows:
   a. Bigeminy
   b. Trigeminy
   c. Constrictive physiology
   d. Kussmaul's sign
   e. Pulsus paradoxus

A transthoracic echocardiogram confirmed the presence of a large pericardial effusion with right atrial (RA) and right ventricular (RV) diastolic collapse. There was marked respiratory variation in the aortic and mitral valve velocities.

2. What is the most likely diagnosis associated with the RA pressure waveforms shown on Figure 8.2?
   a. RV infarction
   b. Tricuspid regurgitation
   c. Congestive heart failure
   d. Pericardial constriction
   e. Tamponade

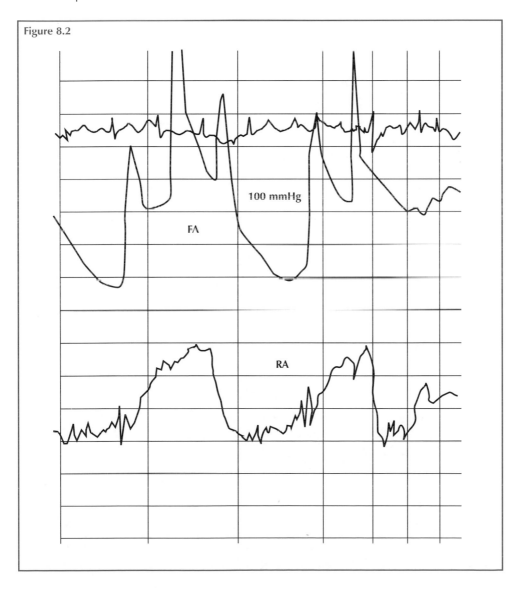

Figure 8.2

Pulmonary artery and RV systolic pressures were recorded. RV pressure was 62/20 mmHg, pulmonary artery pressure was 64/40 mmHg and mean pulmonary artery pressure was 48 mmHg (Figure 8.3). Mean RA and mean pericardial pressures were equal at 40 mmHg (Figure 8.4).

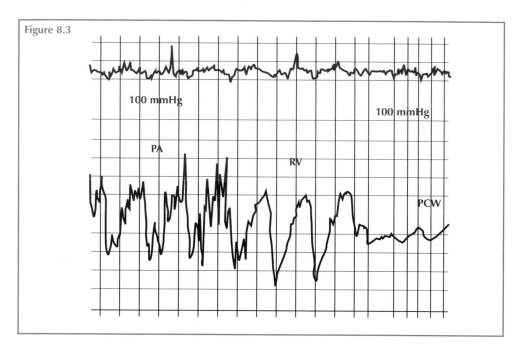

Figure 8.3

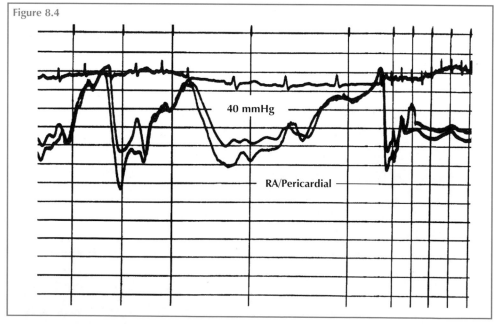

Figure 8.4

Pericardiocentesis for tamponade was performed. After removal of 1450 mL of fluid, both pericardial and RA pressures decreased (Figure 8.5). Echocardiography demonstrated complete resolution of the pericardial effusion.

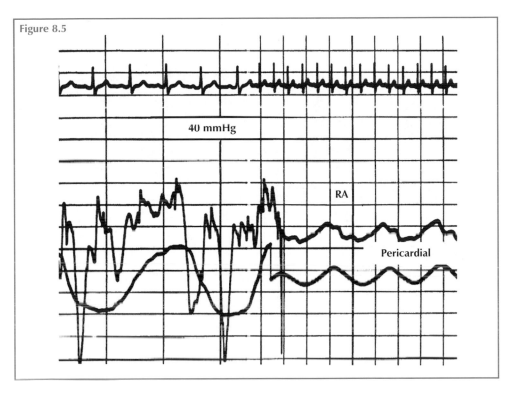

Figure 8.5

3. Following pericardiocentesis (Figure 8.6), what processes explain why pericardial pressure does not return to zero?
   a. RV perforation
   b. RA perforation
   c. Constrictive pericarditis
   d. Effusive constrictive pericardial restraint
   e. Incomplete fluid removal

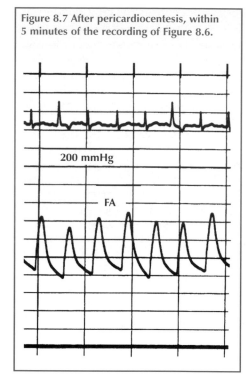

Figure 8.6 Restoration of phasic RV waveform after pericardiocentesis. Exaggerated respiratory variations persist.

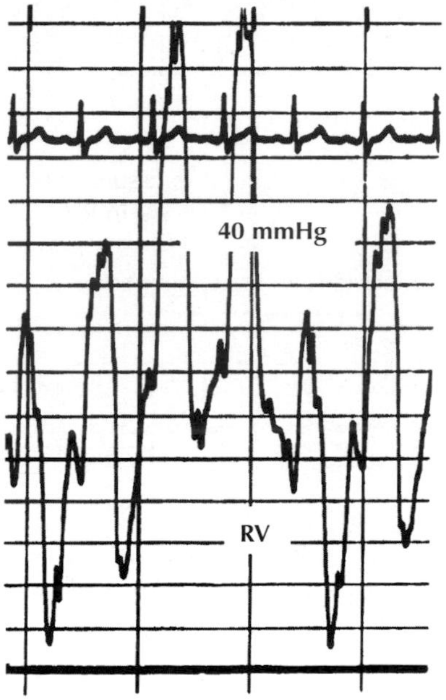

40 mmHg

RV

Figure 8.7 After pericardiocentesis, within 5 minutes of the recording of Figure 8.6.

200 mmHg

FA

4. **After pericardiocentesis, the arterial pressure is recorded again (Figure 8.7). This tracing shows:**
   a. Atrial fibrillation
   b. Constrictive physiology
   c. Pulsus paradoxus
   d. Pre-tamponade pulse pressure
   e. Normal pressure waveform

Answers

1. e Pulsus paradoxus is an increased inspiratory decline (>10–15 mmHg) in arterial systolic pressure, which may obliterate the arterial waveform at the end of inspiration. In this case, the average arterial pressure was 120/80 mmHg; however, associated with a pulsus paradoxus of 80 mmHg, the femoral arterial pulse was completely lost during inspiration, giving an appearance of grouped beating.

Inspiration causes a decrease in intrathoracic, intrapericardial and RA pressure, resulting in augmented flow from the vena cava into the RA and a marked increase in RV volume. There is a decrease in left ventricular (LV) filling pressures and volume, resulting from a septal displacement from right to left, accompanied by a decrease in the aortic flow and systolic arterial pressure. Pulsus paradoxus can be detected by a decrease in the amplitude of the palpated femoral or carotid pulse during inspiration. It can be quantified by cuff sphygmomanometry and auscultation by determining the difference in pressure when the Korotkoff sounds are heard only during expiration and when they are heard equally during both expiration and inspiration. A pulsus paradoxus of <10 mmHg is normal.

Kussmaul's sign reflects an increase in systemic venous pressure (or at least the absence of a decrease) with inspiration, reflecting the inability of negative intrathoracic pressures to be transmitted to the pericardial space of cardiac chambers, as seen with constrictive pericarditis.

Claude S Beck (1935) described the triad of findings that occur with cardiac tamponade following sudden intrapericardial hemorrhage (abrupt addition of 200 mL of blood/fluid to a non-stretched pericardium):
1. decline in systemic arterial pressure
2. elevation of systemic venous pressure
3. a small quiet heart.

Clinically, the most common physical finding is an elevated jugular venous pressure with a characteristic waveform demonstrating a prominent X-descent with an absent diastolic Y-descent. Other characteristic findings in patients with tamponade include tachypnea (80%), tachycardia (77%), pulsus paradoxus (77%), pericardial friction rub and diminished heart sounds.

2. e Cardiac tamponade is characterized by elevation of intracardiac pressures, progressive limitation of ventricular diastolic filling and reduction of stroke volume and cardiac output. Tamponade occurs when the intrapericardial pressure equalizes with the ventricular filling pressures, resulting in a markedly diminished transmural distending pressure (ventricular end-diastolic pressure minus pericardial pressure) and a subsequent reduction in the ventricular end-diastolic volume and stroke volume. Venous return is also reduced as the intrapericardial pressure increases and becomes equal to or exceeds the RA diastolic pressure. This mechanism limits the systemic venous surge and reduces phasic atrial pressure waves. As the tricuspid valve opens, RA emptying is impeded. This is manifested graphically as an absent or attenuated Y-descent during right heart catheterization.

The RA waveform is elevated with a mean of 40 mmHg. In addition, the narrow systemic pulse pressure and tachycardia are indicative of reduced cardiac output. The RA waveform is also usual in the obliteration of its phasic components. Respiratory variation in pressure is marked and coincides with loss of arterial pressure during inspiration.

3. **d** Successful relief of cardiac tamponade is documented by:
   1. the fall of intrapericardial pressures to levels between −3 and +3 mmHg
   2. the fall of an elevated RA pressure, with separation of simultaneous right and left heart filling pressures
   3. increased cardiac output
   4. disappearance of pulsus paradoxus.

The presence of continued elevation and equilibration of right and left filling pressures with the appearance of a prominent Y-descent in RA pressure strongly suggest the presence of a constricting pericardium due to effusive-constrictive pericarditis. In this case, only partial resolution was seen (by echocardiography) following complete pericardiocentesis.

4. **e** The arterial pulse is restored, with only the normal 10–15 mmHg inspiratory decline in systolic pressure, eliminating the dramatic pulsus paradoxus.

Chapter 9
Constriction/Restriction

A 31-year-old woman with pulmonary sarcoidosis presents with 6 months of fatigue and increasing positional chest discomfort, worse when supine. A three-component friction rub is appreciated. Right heart catheterization is performed. The right atrial (RA) and right ventricular (RV) pressures are recorded at rest with a fluid-filled catheter (Figure 9.1).

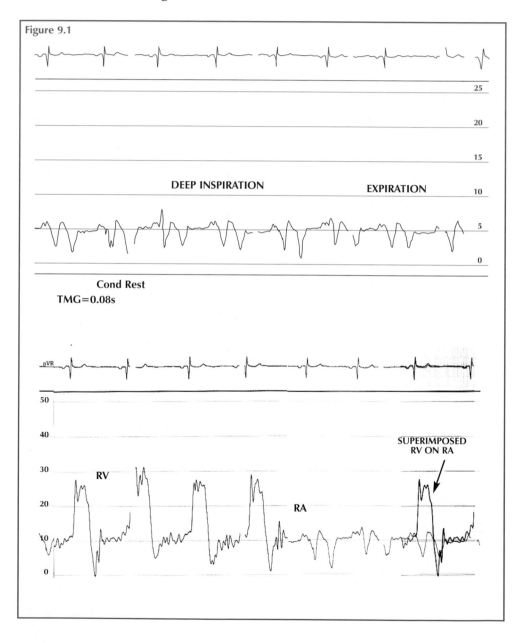

Figure 9.1

1. Which of the following does the RA pressure tracing in Figure 9.1 demonstrate?
   a. Elevated RA pressure
   b. Normal RA hemodynamics
   c. Kussmaul's sign
   d. Exaggerated X- and Y-descents
   e. Both (c) and (d) are correct

2. The RA and RV hemodynamics in this patient suggest a diagnosis of:
   a. RV infarction
   b. Pericardial tamponade
   c. Tricuspid stenosis
   d. Pericardial constriction
   e. The hemodynamic and physical findings are non-specific

3. Classic hemodynamic findings are not always present in patients with pericardial constriction. Which of the following hemodynamic maneuvers can uncover occult constriction?
   a. Dobutamine infusion
   b. Valsalva's maneuver
   c. Rapid saline infusion
   d. Phenylephrine infusion
   e. Nitroglycerin infusion

A 37-year-old woman with prior viral illness presents with increasing dyspnea on exertion. Hemodynamics are shown in Figures 9.2a and 9.2b.

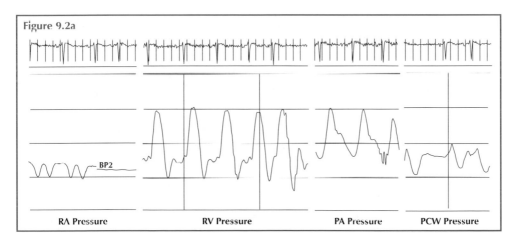

Figure 9.2a

RA Pressure   RV Pressure   PA Pressure   PCW Pressure

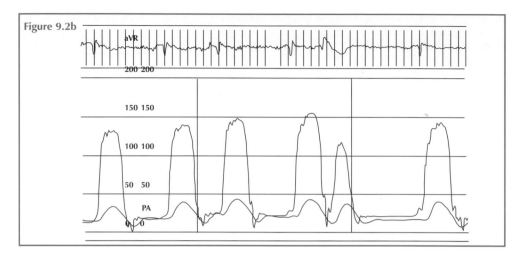

Figure 9.2b

4. **What is the most likely diagnosis based on the hemodynamic tracings in Figure 9.2?**
   a. Congestive heart failure
   b. Mitral regurgitation
   c. Chronic pericarditis
   d. Cardiac tamponade
   e. Pulmonary stenosis

5. **This hemodynamic tracing (Figure 9.3) most clearly demonstrates:**
   a. Tamponade
   b. Congestive heart failure
   c. Restrictive cardiomyopathy
   d. Pericardial constriction
   e. Tricuspid regurgitation

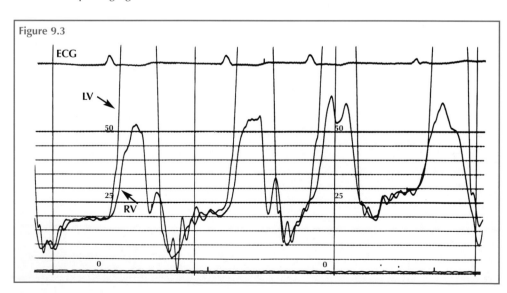

Figure 9.3

6. The diagnosis suspected in Figure 9.3 may be confirmed with which of the following maneuvers?
   a. Handgrip
   b. Valsalva maneuver
   c. Rapid saline infusion
   d. Examination of normal respiratory LV/RV systolic pressure relationship
   e. Squatting

7. In a patient with dyspnea on exertion, this hemodynamic tracing (Figure 9.4) is most likely associated with:
   a. Tamponade
   b. Congestive heart failure
   c. Mitral stenosis
   d. Pericardial constriction
   e. Myocardial restriction

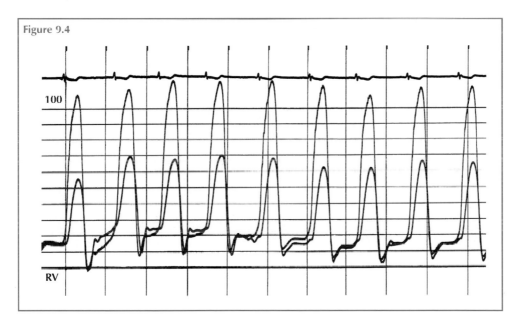

Figure 9.4

A 60-year-old woman from eastern Europe presents with cough, weight loss and dyspnea at rest. Her chest x-ray (Figure 9.5) and hemodynamics (Figures 9.6 and 9.7) are shown.

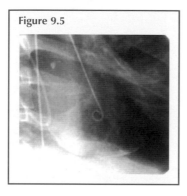

Figure 9.5

8. Which of the following is the most likely cause of the clinical syndrome (Figure 9.5) and hemodynamic tracings (Figures 9.6 and 9.7)?
   a. Viral pericarditis
   b. Tubercular pericarditis
   c. Pericardial sarcoidosis
   d. Trauma with pneumopericardium
   e. Malignant melanoma of pericardium

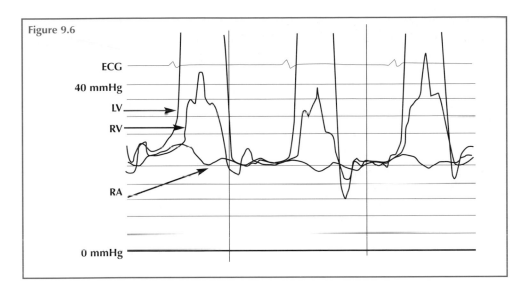

Figure 9.6

ECG
40 mmHg
LV
RV
RA
0 mmHg

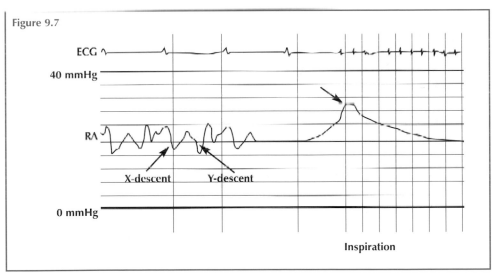

Figure 9.7

ECG
40 mmHg
RA
X-descent   Y-descent
0 mmHg
Inspiration

Answers

1. **e** Kussmaul's sign is defined as a rise in, or failure to decrease, RA pressure with inspiration. In this case, RA pressure fails to decline during inspiration, a response that is always abnormal in the absence of positive pressure (mechanical) ventilation. The X- and Y-descents are also exaggerated. The Y-descent is greater than the X-descent during inspiration. The RV tracing demonstrates a 'dip and plateau' or 'square root' sign. Note that in the superimposed RV beat, the 'dip' corresponds to the Y-descent.

2. **d** The 'square root' sign and deep Y-descent are characteristic of the rapid diastolic pressure rise (and equilibration) from pericardial constraint. Kussmaul's sign occurs in pericardial constriction, RV dysfunction and occasionally with tricuspid stenosis. It is not associated with pericardial tamponade. Tamponade is often associated with blunted X- and Y-descents and higher RA and RV end-diastolic pressures. Tricuspid stenosis is typically associated with elevated mean RA pressure and a large A-wave. RV infarction may have a pattern of constriction and is also associated with an elevated RVEDP. In the presence of acute inferior infarction, Kussmaul's sign is highly accurate for detecting RV involvement.

3. **c** Patients with low right heart filling pressures may have relative volume depletion and not manifest the expected findings of pericardial constraint. Some patients may develop 'low-pressure' tamponade, and manifest weakness and exertional dyspnea in the absence of jugular venous distension or pulsus paradoxus. Diastolic pressures may equalize only during inspiration. Rapid volume loading with a saline infusion (or by passively elevating the legs) may abruptly elevate RA pressure and produce persistent diastolic pressure equalization and pulsus paradoxus. Although not diagnostic, exercise can also elevate RA pressure, probably as a consequence of augmented venous return. In this patient, RA pressure is elevated already at 12 mmHg (bottom tracing).

4. **c** Constrictive pericardial pathophysiology is characterized by near-equalization of all diastolic chamber and venous pressures, a 'square root' configuration of RV and LV diastolic tracings, an RVEDP that is at least one-third of the RV systolic pressure, and an RA pressure tracing Y-descent nadir equal to or greater than the X-descent. Tamponade physiology typically manifests as an elevated RA pressure with an absent or decreased Y-descent and exaggerated respiratory pressure changes (including the systemic arterial pulsus paradoxus).

5. **d** Restrictive cardiomyopathy typically demonstrates a discordance in LV/RV diastolic pressures with LVEDP > RVEDP by >5 mmHg, which can be further accentuated by exercise, fluid challenge and the Valsalva maneuver. This is probably due to the predominant effect of restriction on the more muscular LV as compared to the more compliant RV. In this respect, restriction differs from constrictive pericarditis, where diastolic pressures are equalized between both ventricles due to extrinsic compression (usually RV/LV diastolic pressures differ by <5 mmHg).

The plateau of the RV diastolic pressures in this case also exceeds 30% of RV systolic pressures, which is suggestive of constrictive pericarditis.

However, up to one in four patients may still need exploratory thoracotomy with pericardial stripping and myocardial biopsy for definitive diagnosis, as classification cannot be made on hemodynamic grounds.

The differentiation between restriction and constriction is mandatory because of the potential for successful surgical treatment of constriction.

6. d Normal inspiration can yield information differentiating constrictive from restrictive physiology. Concordance of LV/RV systolic pressures is more sensitive for diagnosis of restrictive cardiomyopathy, whereas respiratory discordance is highly consistent for constrictive pericarditis (Figure 9.8).

Figure 9.8

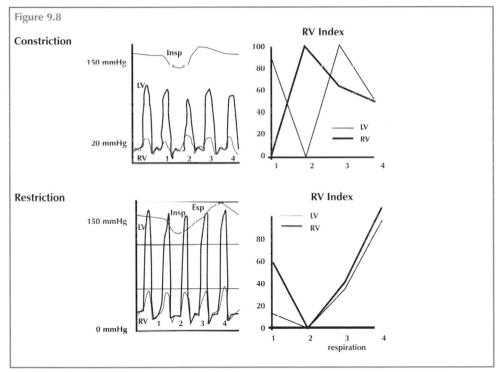

Reproduced with permission from Hurrell DG. Value of dynamic respiratory changes in left and right ventricular pressures for the diagnosis of constrictive pericarditis. Circulation 1996;93:2007–13.

7.   e Controlled respiration, the simplest maneuver, can differentiate tamponade physiology from constriction via the pulsus paradoxus and Kussmaul's sign. The increased venous return during inspiration may also deepen the nadir of the Y-descent and the diastolic 'dip' on the ventricular pressure tracing (see Table 9.1).

Table 9.1 Sensitivities, specificities, positive predictive value and negative predictive value as a function of criteria for the diagnosis of constrictive pericarditis.

Criteria	Sensitivity (%)	Specificity (%)	PPV (%)	NPV (%)
Conventional				
LVEDP–RVEDP <5 mmHg	60	38	4	57
RVEDP/RVSP >1/3	93	38	52	89
PASP <55 mmHg	93	24	47	25
LV RFW ≤7 mmHg	93	57	61	92
Respiratory change RAP <3 mmHg	93	48	58	92
Dynamic respiratory				
PCWP/LV respiratory gradient ≤5 mmHg	93	81	78	94
LV/RV interdependence	100	95	94	100

(Reproduced with permission from Hurrell DG. Value of dynamic respiratory changes in left and right ventricular pressures for the diagnosis of constrictive pericarditis. Circulation 1996;93:2007–13.)

LV: left ventricular; LVEDP: left ventricular end-diastolic pressure; NPV: negative predictive value; PASP: pulmonary artery systolic pressure; PCWP: pulmonary capillary wedge pressure; PPV: positive predictive value; RAP: right atrial pressure; RFW: rapid filling wave; RV: right ventricular; RVEDP: right ventricular end-diastolic pressure; RVSP: right ventricular systolic pressure.

8.   b A calcified pericardial shell is most commonly associated with tuberculosis. Other conditions such as hemorrhage or trauma may cause pericardial calcification after many years.

Chapter 10
Atrial Septal Defects

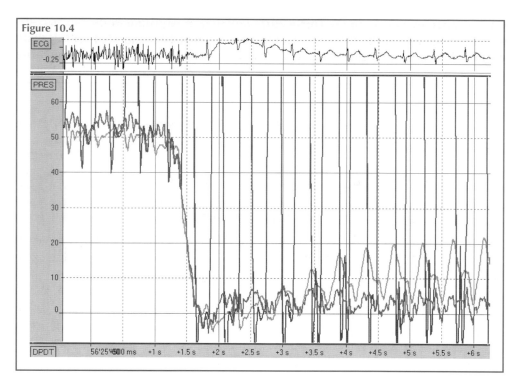

Figure 10.4

2. From the hemodynamic responses to the maneuver performed in Figures 10.2, 10.3 and 10.4, which of the following best describes the pressure changes during the maneuver? (Hint: examine Figures 10.3 and 10.4 closely.)

a. Decreased arterial pulse pressure
b. RA > LA pressure
c. LA > RA pressure
d. LA < left ventricular end-diastolic pressure (LVEDP)
e. RA < LVEDP

A 72-year-old woman has hypotension and refractory hypoxia in the intensive care unit (ICU). RA and LA pressures are measured on continuous catheter pullback (LA to RA), following transseptal catheterization (Figure 10.5).

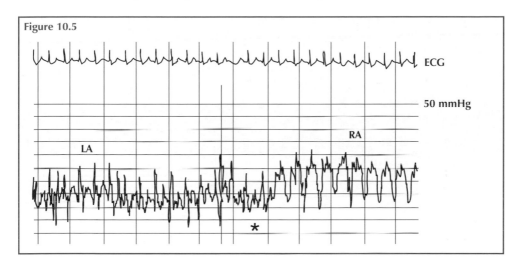

Figure 10.5

3. What is the anatomic etiology of this patient's hypoxia?
    a. Atrioventricular canal defect
    b. Pulmonary hypertension
    c. Patent foramen ovale (PFO)
    d. Truncus arteriosus with aortic (Ao)–pulmonary artery (PA) window
    e. Tricuspid regurgitation

4. Which physiologic cause of this patient's hypoxia is demonstrated?
    a. Arteriovenous shunting due to pulmonary fistulae
    b. Pulmonary embolus
    c. Left-to-right shunting due to ventricular septal defect (VSD)
    d. Right-to-left shunting due to VSD
    e. Right-to-left shunting due to atrial septal defect (ASD)

5. On Figure 10.5, why is the RA pressure higher than the LA pressure?
    a. Artifact
    b. Acute LV infarction
    c. Chronic LV failure
    d. Ebstein's anomaly
    e. Acute RV infarction

6. A 32-year-old patient, with a known ostium secundum ASD with left-to-right shunting shown previously by echocardiography, is taken to the catheterization laboratory. Which is the correct calculated value of the Qp:Qs shunt ratio?

SVC O$_2$ sat = 50%
IVC O$_2$ sat = 60%
RV O$_2$ sat = 68%
RA O$_2$ sat = 66%
PA O$_2$ sat = 72%
FA O$_2$ sat = 96%
Hb = 12 g/dL
F$_i$O$_2$ = 21%
O$_2$ consumption = 200 mL/min

FA: femoral artery; Hb: hemoglobin; IVC: inferior vena cava; PA: pulmonary artery; RA: right atrium; RV: right ventricle; SVC: superior vena cava.

   a. 1.25:1.0
   b. 1.5:1.0
   c. 1.7:1.0
   d. 1.8:1.0
   e. 2.0:1.0

7. What therapeutic recommendation would you make for this patient?
   a. Daily aspirin to reduce risk of cerebrovascular accident
   b. Conservative management with observation, because Qp:Qs > 1.5:1.0
   c. Conservative management with observation, because Qp:Qs < 1.5:1.0
   d. Operative management, either open or percutaneous, because Qp:Qs > 1.5:1.0
   e. Subacute bacterial endocarditis prophylaxis

Answers

1. **a3, b2, c1**

    LA pressure normally exceeds RA pressures when only a small ASD or PFO is present, whereas the mean pressures in both atria are nearly equal when the ASD is large. Left-to-right shunting occurs predominantly in late ventricular systole and early diastole with some augmentation during atrial contraction. The magnitude of left-to-right shunting depends on the size of the ASD and the relative compliance of the ventricles, and the relative resistance in both the pulmonary and systemic circulations.

2. **b** These hemodynamics demonstrate that RA pressure increases above LA pressure during the Valsalva maneuver in a patient with PFO. Therefore, paradoxic embolization may occur in patients during straining or other everyday activities. At times, a PFO may exhibit paroxysmal right-to-left shunting. The systolic pressure falls during the Valsalva maneuver (as shown on LV tracing, the peripheral arterial pulse is not shown on this tracing).

3. **c** A pressure gradient is seen with RA pressures being greater than LA. Chronic pulmonary hypertension is likely to present, causing the elevated central venous pressure, although pulmonary hypertension alone is not causative of systemic hypoxia. The atrial septal defect is small (i.e. a restrictive PFO), as RA and LA pressures are commonly equalized in patients with a larger ASD.

    Cyanosis with significant mixing of blood could result from a truncus arteriosus defect, but such a patient would be very unlikely to survive into late adulthood given the significant morbidity and mortality in very early life. Similarly, AV canal defects usually are large enough to provide equalization of RA and LA pressures. There are no prominent V-waves on the RA tracing to suggest tricuspid regurgitation.

4. **e** Desaturated venous blood is shunted from the RA to the LA via the PFO when RV pressure increases RA pressure dramatically. Although answers (a) and (b) are clinically possible, they cannot be diagnosed from the data provided.

5. **e** RV infarction increases RV and RA pressures and, in the presence of a PFO, can result in right-to-left shunting.

    RV infarction patients often present with hypotension, clear lungs and low pulmonary capillary wedge (PCW) pressure. RV pressure waveforms also appear similar to that of constrictive physiology with dip and plateau configuration.

A tamponading balloon placed across the PFO (to eliminate shunting) has been used in severely ill patients to improve oxygenation (Figure 10.6).

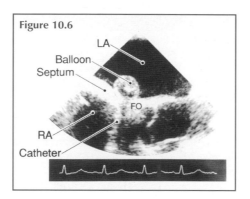

Figure 10.6

LA
Balloon
Septum
FO
RA
Catheter

In adulthood, Ebstein's anomaly (apical displacement of the tricuspid valve) is not usually associated with an elevated RA pressure, although significant tricuspid regurgitation may occur. LA pressures are usually elevated in the setting of acute LV myocardial infarction.

6.   d The Fick method principles for determining cardiac output are used to quantify intracardiac shunts. Pulmonary and systemic blood flow determinations are required to determine the size of the shunt. Pulmonary blood flow (Qp) and systemic blood flow (Qs) are simply the oxygen consumption divided by the difference in O_2 content across the pulmonary or systemic bed, respectively.

$$Qp = \frac{O_2 \text{ consumption (mL/min)}}{PVO_2 - PAO_2}; \qquad Qs = \frac{O_2 \text{ consumption (mL/min)}}{SAO_2 - MVO_2}$$

If a pulmonary vein is not sampled, systemic arterial (SA) O_2 content can be substituted, provided arterial saturation is ≥95%. The Flamm formula provides the arterial venous oxygen content (as direct RA measurements are unreliable in ASD patients). MVO_2 is the abbreviation for mixed venous oxygen content.

$$MVO_2 = \frac{3 \text{ (SVC } O_2 \text{ content)} + 1 \text{ (IVC } O_2 \text{ content)}}{4}$$

Rearranging: $\dfrac{Qp}{Qs} = \dfrac{SAO_2 - MVO_2}{PVO_2 - PAO_2}$

$$= \frac{96 - 52.5}{96 - 72} = \frac{43.5}{24} = 1.8$$

Therefore Qp:Qs = 1.8:1.0

7.   d This patient with a Qp:Qs of 1.8:1.0 is a candidate for closure of the secundum ASD. Early surgical repair is definitive with a surgical mortality of <1%. Transcatheter clam-shell or buttoned devices are used increasingly in an effort to avoid morbidity associated with thoracotomy. SBE prophylaxis therapy is not required in isolated secundum ASD, as the risk of infective endocarditis is negligible.

Chapter 11
Congenital Heart Disease

6. In relation to anomalies associated with tetralogy of Fallot, which of the following statements is true?
   a. PFO or small ASD is uncommon
   b. When discovered in infancy, associated coronary anomalies may lead to a decision to postpone definitive surgical repair
   c. Pulmonary valve anomalies are rare because the obstruction is mainly subvalvular
   d. There is a mitral-aortic valve discontinuity
   e. The aortic arch is right-sided in >80% of cases

7. Regarding the physiology of tetralogy of Fallot, which of the following statements is true?
   a. Commonly, there is a gradient between RV and left ventricular (LV) pressures secondary to restrictive VSD
   b. The magnitude and direction of the shunt depends on the size of VSD
   c. Iron-deficiency anemia places individuals with tetralogy of Fallot at risk for cerebrovascular events
   d. Systemic-to-pulmonary artery collateral circulation is extremely rare in tetralogy of Fallot
   e. Thrombocytosis is rare

8. The severity of PS in tetralogy of Fallot determines all of the following, except:
   a. The severity of cyanosis
   b. The degree of hypoxemia
   c. The magnitude of right-to-left shunt
   d. Single S_2 in severe PS, and a split S_2 in mild PS
   e. With increasing severity, the systolic murmur is longer and peaks later

9. After surgical repair of tetralogy of Fallot, which of the following is associated with the poorest outcome:
   a. Right ventricular systolic pressure (RVSP) ≥60 mmHg
   b. Residual VSD with a Qp:Qs of ≥1.5:1
   c. Pulmonary arterial hypertension (distal pulmonary artery pressure (PAP) ≥40 mmHg)
   d. Pulmonary regurgitation
   e. Left ventricular outflow tract (LVOT) obstruction

Answers

1. **c** The simultaneous hemodynamic and intracardiac electrocardiographic recordings (from a catheter tip sensor) during catheter pullback from the RV into the RA reveal the characteristic 'atrialization' of the RV, consistent with Ebstein's anomaly. This is manifested by the presence of an RV electrocardiogram (ECG) simultaneously recorded with RA pressures. With continuing pullback into the RA, the morphology of the ECG signal converts; the P-wave amplitude is exaggerated consistent with an atrial signal, and the QRS amplitude is reduced suggesting a loss of ventricular voltage as the sensor tip is withdrawn further from the RV.

    The major congenital abnormality in Ebstein's anomaly is an apical displacement of the tricuspid valve into the RV, due to anomalous attachment of the tricuspid leaflets away from the atrioventricular junction. This produces an 'atrialized' portion of the RV above and a small RV below, which often has a reduced contractile capability and significantly reduced chamber volume. The degree of RV systolic function impairment is also dependent upon the magnitude of tricuspid valve regurgitation and structural obstruction to RV inflow or outflow. Case control studies suggest that maternal ingestion of lithium carbonate during the first trimester may be associated with an increased incidence of Ebstein's anomaly.

    Since the advent of 2-dimensional (2 D) and Doppler ultrasound, echocardiography has become the diagnostic tool of choice to identify this anomaly. The principal findings in adults include tricuspid regurgitation, RV volume overload, paradoxical ventricular septal motion, an increased tricuspid valve excursion and a delayed closing velocity of the tricuspid leaflets when compared to the mitral valve. Specific diagnosis requires the 2-D identification of displaced septal and posterior tricuspid leaflets in the apical 4-chamber view. A resting 12-lead ECG usually reveals RA enlargement with tall P waves that may be the largest of any syndrome (Himalayan P-waves), PR interval prolongation, frequent right bundle branch block and ventricular depolarization abnormalities. Prior to the advent of echocardiography, cardiac catheterization was required to demonstrate hemodynamic findings and image the displaced tricuspid leaflets during right ventriculography.

2. **c** The tricuspid valve leaflet attachments are ventricularly displaced (towards the ventricular apex), resulting in an anatomically enlarged RA and small RV chamber. Pulmonic valve stenosis, or atresia, is a commonly associated congenital defect, but is not characteristic of Ebstein's anomaly. The mitral valve usually is anatomically normal.

    An interatrial communication, either PFO or secundum ASD, is present in more than 50% of cases, resulting in a right-to-left interatrial shunt. An ostium primum ASD or VSD may also occur in isolation or in combination with other lesions. The most common associated congenital defect is pulmonic valve stenosis or atresia. Ebstein's anomaly is commonly associated with congenitally corrected transposition of the great arteries, in which the tricuspid valve is in the left atrioventricular orifice.

3. **c** Ebstein's anomaly is compatible with a long and active life. Most patients survive into the third decade. During infancy, cyanosis and congestive heart failure are common and may be suddenly intensified as pulmonary hypoperfusion is unmasked by spontaneous closure of a patent ductus arteriosus. Tricuspid regurgitation in the neonate is enhanced

because the pulmonary vascular resistance is normally high early in life. The tricuspid regurgitation seen in infants may lessen substantially, and cyanosis may disappear early in life as pulmonary vascular resistance falls, only to recur at a later age with the development of RV dysfunction or paroxysmal arrhythmias. Beyond infancy, the onset of symptoms is insidious; the most common complaints are exertional dyspnea, fatigue or cyanosis.

4.　c　Accessory atrioventricular conduction pathways are found in 25% or more of patients with Ebstein's anomaly, classically resulting in paroxysmal atrioventricular re-entrant tachycardia. If life-threatening arrhythmias occur, the accessory pathways should be ablated. Atrial fibrillation and flutter occur to a lesser degree. Ventricular tachycardia with left bundle branch block contour with right axis deviation and T-wave inversion in the right precordial leads is associated with RV (arrhythmogenic) dysplasia. Wolff-Parkinson-White 'pattern' is an electrocardiographic description only, whereas Wolff-Parkinson-White 'syndrome' is associated with a tachyarrhythmia.

The primary goals for treatment of Ebstein's anomaly are management of heart failure, prevention of endocarditis, and prevention and treatment of arrhythmias. The results of surgery are unpredictable, with mortality following tricuspid valve replacement reaching 10–15%. Therefore, valvular reconstruction is preferred, if possible.

5.　b　Fallot originally described the tetralogy as consisting of:
1. perimembranous VSD
2. PS
3. the aorta overriding the ventricular septum
4. RV hypertrophy.

The associated anomalies of tetralogy of Fallot (TOF) include ASD or PFO in 50% of patients, AV canal defects in patients with Down syndrome and, rarely, a persistent left superior vena cava that drains directly to the LA. High-risk disorders include anomalous origin of the left anterior descending artery from the right coronary ostia, or a single coronary artery with a major branch crossing the right ventricular outflow tract (RVOT) region (potentially complicating surgical repair).

The major hemodynamic features include a pressure gradient across the infundibular RVOT and equalization of the ventricular pressures secondary to a non-restrictive VSD. Of note, the contour of the RV pressure resembles that of the LV. In cases of PS with intact ventricular septum, there is no equalization of ventricular pressures. However, patients with both VSD and pulmonary hypertension (Eisenmenger's physiology) may exhibit no pressure gradient across the RVOT.

6.　b　The presence of a large coronary artery traversing the RVOT makes surgical relief of sub-valvular PS difficult and introduces substantial risk of myocardial infarction, particularly if an outflow patch is necessary. In this subgroup, surgery will be safer in older and larger patients. Fifty percent of the patients have either a PFO or an ASD.

The pulmonic valve is abnormal in most cases of TOF. Abnormalities include a bicuspid or unicuspid valve that occasionally represents the only site of obstruction to RV outflow (i.e. no infundibular stenosis).

In TOF patients, there is mitral-aortic continuity with the non-coronary and left coronary leaflets in continuous contact with the anterior mitral leaflets. The aortic arch is right-sided in about 20% of the patients. The standard Blalock-Taussig shunt is constructed on the opposite side of the aortic arch because the presence of the innominate artery makes kinking of the anastomosis less likely.

The clinical spectrum of TOF is widely variable. It ranges from the distressed, cyanotic, hypoxemic neonate to the young adult with no cyanosis and few symptoms, depending on the severity of PS.

Cardiac catheterization is not routinely performed before surgical intervention, but oximetry can be used to calculate the pulmonary-to-systemic flow ratio. In 'pink' allot, the pulmonary flow is greater than the systemic flow. The reverse is true in the typical TOF patient. Angiography is superior to echocardiography in regard to detailing the pulmonary arterial tree, detecting coronary anomalies and mapping collateral flow to the lungs.

7. c Polycythemia alters blood coagulation; deficiency of one or more coagulation factors is common if the hematocrit exceeds 65%. Very high hematocrit levels, or iron deficiency with resultant microcytosis, increases blood viscosity and places patients at higher risk for cerebrovascular events. The VSD is usually large and non-restrictive, resulting in equal peak systolic pressures in the two ventricles. The magnitude and direction of the flow through the defect depend more on the severity of PS. Moderate PS is associated with left-to-right shunt at the ventricular level. However, a severely stenotic pulmonary valve is associated with more right-to-left shunting.

An extensive systemic-to-pulmonary collateral circulation is more characteristic of TOF associated with pulmonary artery atresia than with PS.

8. e The VSD is silent to auscultation in TOF, but its presence modifies the murmur of PS. When the ventricular septum is intact, the murmur tends to be louder, longer and later peaking with severe obstruction. The opposite occurs when PS coexists with VSD. As PS becomes more severe, the volume of the right-to-left shunt increases and less blood traverses the RVOT, so the murmur is softer.

If the PS obstruction is more severe, the degree of right-to-left shunting is increased and more unsaturated blood will enter the aorta, resulting in more severe cyanosis. In patients with mild TOF, cyanosis will be absent and loud systolic murmur will be heard over the left sternal border. The presence of RV hypertrophy by electrocardiography together with right-sided aortic arch on chest x-ray suggests the possibility of TOF.

The second heart sound is always single if there is cyanosis, since severe PS results in low pulmonary artery pressure, making the pulmonic closure sound inaudible.

9. **e** LVOT obstruction is rare following TOF surgical repair, and may be related to a complicated patch closure of the large VSD. There is usually at least some degree of RV outflow obstruction following surgery. Pulmonary regurgitation is present in the majority of cases, but most agree that even major pulmonary regurgitation is well tolerated for many years. However, the combination of pulmonary regurgitation and residual RV hypertension (secondary to residual outflow obstruction or residual VSD) is associated with a poorer prognosis.

Surgical treatment is indicated if the patient has a decreased exercise tolerance, hypercyanotic spells, excessively high hemoglobin or if the patient has attained the appropriate size and age for repair. Palliative shunts are considered when patients are not considered good candidates for repair. Percutaneous balloon dilatation of the RVOT has been used as an alternative method of palliation, but intracardiac repair remains the ideal treatment. The ideal age for surgical repair is under debate. The presence of high-risk coronary anomalies might be a good reason to postpone surgery. Common causes of re-operation include residual VSD, PS or pulmonary regurgitation. Sudden death is a recognized complication, and is more prevalent in patients with hemodynamic abnormalities.

Chapter 12

Arrhythmias

A 66-year-old man presents with an acute myocardial infarction and is successfully treated with thrombolytics. On hospital day three, there is a sudden mild decrease in arterial pressure. A change in his rhythm is noted on telemetry. The right atrial (RA) pressure waveform is shown on Figure 12.1.

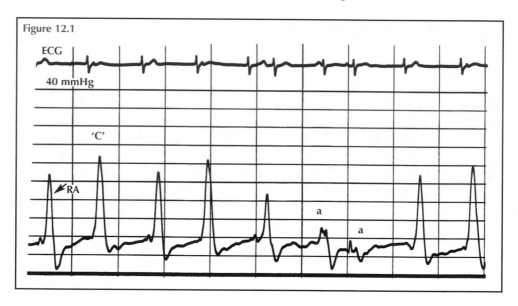

Figure 12.1

1. **What is the cardiac rhythm?**
   a. Atrial fibrillation
   b. Wandering atrial pacemaker
   c. Junctional rhythm with high-grade atrioventricular (AV) block
   d. Atrial bigeminy
   e. Sinus rhythm with frequent premature atrial contractions

2. **What are the symptoms most likely to be experienced by a patient with this hemodynamic presentation?**
   a. Palpitations
   b. Syncope
   c. Fullness in the neck
   d. Yellow or green visual halo
   e. No symptoms are typical

3. **What finding, on physical examination, correlates with this hemodynamic presentation?**
   a. Absence of an S_4
   b. Irregular large pulsatile jugular venous waves
   c. Parasternal heave
   d. Kussmaul's sign
   e. Pulsatile liver

4. **What phenomenon explains the change in waveform morphology in the beats labeled 'a'?**
   a. AV dyssynchrony
   b. AV synchrony
   c. Respiratory variation
   d. Valsalva maneuver
   e. Pacemaker rhythm

A 65-year-old hypertensive man with a VVI pacemaker (for sick sinus syndrome) presents with intermittent fatigue and presyncope. Left ventricular (LV) and aortic (Ao) pressures are recorded at catheterization (Figure 12.2).

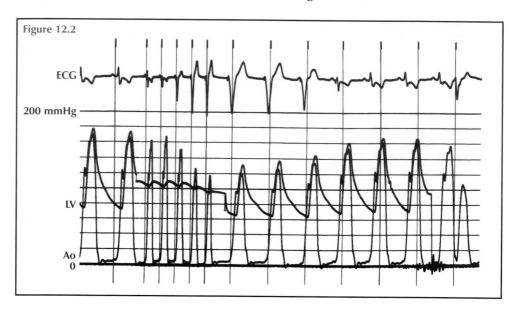

Figure 12.2

5. The 'pacemaker' syndrome would be most commonly associated with which of the following chronic pacing modes?
   a. VVI
   b. AAI
   c. DDD
   d. DDDR
   e. AAT

6. The hemodynamic effects of AV dissociation include all of the following except:
   a. Reduced stroke volume
   b. Decreased systolic arterial pressure
   c. Decreased pulmonary capillary wedge (PCW) pressure
   d. Increased RA pressure
   e. Reduced LV end-diastolic pressure (LVEDP)

7. Physiologic cardiac pacing may depend upon:
   a. Rate response to exercise
   b. Programmed AV delay
   c. Pacing mode (VVI vs. DDD)
   d. Pacing site (right ventricular [RV] apex vs. outflow tract)
   e. All the above

8. A physical exam finding representative of the hemodynamic effects of AV dissociation with VVI pacing is:
   a. S_3
   b. Pulsus paradoxus
   c. Cannon A-waves
   d. Systolic ejection murmurs
   e. S_4

9. Revision of a VVI pacemaker system to a dual chamber pacemaker system to alleviate pacemaker syndrome would be least appropriate in which of the following clinical settings?
   a. Sick sinus syndrome with symptomatic bradycardia
   b. Complete heart block with chronic atrial fibrillation
   c. Complete heart block with intact VA conduction
   d. Intermittent Mobitz type-II second degree heart block
   e. Intermittent AV block and sinus node dysfunction in a chronotropically incompetent patient and the presence of significant paroxysmal supraventricular tachycardia (PSVT)

10. What is the single best explanation for the fall in RA peak pressure at the asterisk in Figure 12.3?
    a. Termination of ventricular pacing
    b. Onset of atrial fibrillation
    c. Respiratory variation
    d. Gradual resumption of AV association
    e. Dampened pressure transmission

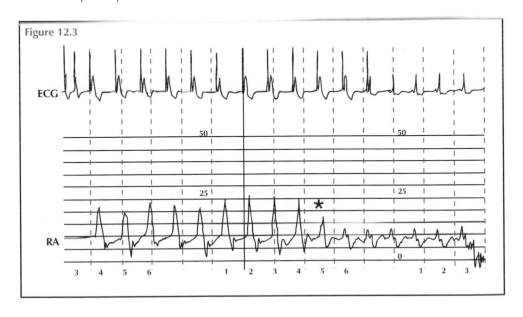

Figure 12.3

A 54-year-old female with insulin-requiring diabetes mellitus presents with decreasing exercise tolerance over the past few years. She has a family history of coronary artery disease, and she recently quit smoking. After evaluation, she was referred for cardiac catheterization. Hemodynamic tracings are shown on Figure 12.4.

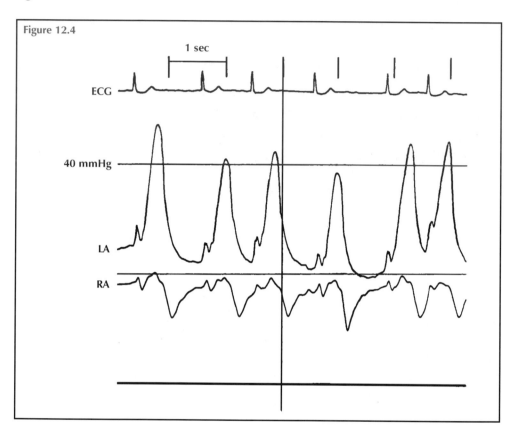

Figure 12.4

11. What is the rhythm?
   a. Atrial fibrillation
   b. Wandering atrial pacemaker
   c. Junctional rhythm with high-grade AV block
   d. Atrial bigeminy
   e. Sinus rhythm with frequent premature atrial contractions

12. What physical exam finding correlates with this tracing?
   a. Absence of an S_4
   b. Kussmaul's sign
   c. Cannon A-waves
   d. Systolic murmur, increasing with respiration
   e. Diastolic murmur, increasing with respiration

13. **Assuming single vessel coronary disease is documented, which coronary distribution would be most likely to account for this tracing?**
    a. Left anterior descending coronary artery
    b. Left circumflex coronary artery
    c. Ramus intermedius coronary artery
    d. Right coronary artery
    e. Cannot determine

14. **The peaked LA waveforms are most consistent with:**
    a. Tricuspid regurgitation
    b. Mitral regurgitation
    c. Ao insufficiency
    d. Mitral stenosis
    e. Tricuspid stenosis

Answers

1. **c** The ECG tracing along the top of the strip demonstrates P-waves that march through the rhythm strip at a constant interval independent of the QRS complexes. The P-wave morphology differs, since some occur during ventricular depolarization while others occur during ventricular repolarization. Cannon A-waves (marked 'C' on the tracing) are recorded when atrial contraction occurs while the tricuspid valve (TV) is closed. When the TV is open, the Cannon A-wave is not seen (beats labeled 'a'), and the pressure waveforms accurately reflect LV filling pressures. Careful study of the ECG and the hemodynamic tracing excludes atrial fibrillation as the rhythm. Note that for the sixth and seventh beats, both A- and V-waves can be distinguished.

2. **c** Atrial dyssynchrony from myocardial ischemia or other causes of high-grade AV block (such as digitalis toxicity or dual-chamber pacing with a failure to track the atria) can result in Cannon A-waves. When atrial systole occurs against a closed tricuspid valve, the blood normally ejected into the ventricle instead refluxes into the jugular veins. Seen as markedly exaggerated A-waves on the RA tracing (Cannon waves), abnormal pulsatile distension of the internal jugular vein is the characteristic finding. This is often perceived as neck fullness by the patient.

    Loss of atrial filling in part explains the 'pacemaker syndrome' experienced by recipients of ventricular pacemakers that do not track atrial activity. Atrial dyssynchrony can result in decreased cardiac output and thus inability to meet metabolic needs during activity, leading to shortness of breath and dyspnea on exertion. Systemic hypotension may also be present, resulting from reduced LV filling due to the loss of an appropriately timed atrial systole.

3. **b** Cannon waves can be transmitted to the jugular veins. Although severe tricuspid regurgitation can be associated with a pulsatile liver, the deflections marked 'C' do not represent giant V-waves (because they are not reliably preceded by a QRS complex). Constrictive pericarditis (Kussmaul's sign) and volume overload (parasternal heave) are expected to reveal distinct Y-descents in the atrial waveform. An intermittent S_4 may be present, representing atrial contraction through an open mitral valve.

4. **b** The hemodynamic and simultaneous ECG tracings demonstrate that the marked beats reflect atrial systole preceding the QRS. In contrast to the other beats, the RA morphology of the beats marked 'a' is normal because the atria are not contracting against a closed tricuspid valve. Fusion beats accentuate the A-waves due to AV dyssynchrony.

    The Valsalva maneuver diminishes both the A-wave and the V-wave by reducing venous return to the RA. Respirophasic variation is normally more gradual in onset (as well as in resolution), and may be expected to alter RA pressures in concert with respiratory activity.

5. **a** Modern cardiac pacing strives to provide physiologic pacing in a variety of pathophysiologic conditions. Pacing mode (VVI, DDD, etc.), timing intervals (AV delay), rate responsiveness and the site of ventricular pacing (RV apex vs. outflow tract) are all-important variables in the provision of physiologic pacing. AV synchrony (the appropriate timing relationship between the mechanical events of atrial and ventricular systole) is the most important tenet of physiologic pacing.

Pacemaker syndrome most commonly occurs when VVI mode is used in patients with sinus rhythm, but it can occur in other modes if AV synchrony is lost. AAI, AAT, DDD and DDDR are all associated with atrial-based pacing, which will minimize the incidence of AV dissociation. AAI and AAT pacing modes (atrium-paced, atrium-sensed, response either inhibited [I] or triggered [T]) both require the intrinsic AV-node to be intact and functional, as there is no ventricular pacemaker activity present. Dual chamber devices are capable of both sensing and pacing in either the atrium or the ventricle, using the sensing information to either inhibit or trigger a response. DDDR pacing mode is dual chamber, with the added benefit of rate responsiveness to a built-in activity or motion sensor.

6. c Figure 12.2 represents the hemodynamic relationship of the Ao and LV pressures during periods of sinus rhythm, as well as a period of ventricular demand pacing. The initial two ECG complexes are sinus rhythm with hypertensive LV and Ao pressures and no transvalvular gradient. The next five ECG complexes demonstrate progressive AV dissociation with onset of ventricular demand pacing (note the transient compression of the tracing time axis: each vertical bar represents one second). The loss of AV synchrony is associated with a profound fall in Ao pressure; in this case, a clear explanation for this patient's intermittent presyncope. AV synchrony returns with the resumption of sinus rhythm and restoration of LV and Ao pressures to near baseline levels.

The loss of coordinated AV activation increases both RA and LA pressures as the tricuspid and mitral valves may be closed during atrial systole. PCW pressure is accordingly increased, not only on the basis of increased A-wave amplitude (reversing pressure to the pulmonary veins) but also as a result of reduced LV forward stroke volume subsequent to reduced LV filling with the loss of a coordinated atrial impulse. LV end-diastolic volumes and pressures are both reduced, shifting the Frank-Starling curve to the left.

The entire spectrum of clinical symptoms associated with loss of AV association is referred to as 'Pacemaker Syndrome'. While common in the era of single chamber ventricular-based pacing, dual chamber and atrial-based single chamber pacemaker systems have reduced the frequency of pacemaker syndrome by maintaining AV synchrony.

The hemodynamic effects of AV dissociation include arterial hypotension, reduced cardiac stroke volume, intraventricular pressure gradients and elevated filling pressures associated with a wide spectrum of signs and symptoms. True syncope from arterial hypotension and pulmonary congestion resulting from reduced cardiac output is uncommon in the typical pacemaker patient population. AV dissociation during chronic cardiac pacing more commonly results in complaints of fatigue, poor exercise tolerance, dyspnea and neck pulsations or fullness.

7. e Rate-responsive systems are designed to mimic true exertional physiology by increasing the programmed (paced) heart rate in response to an electronically-sensed activity or motion stimulus. Pacing mode and programmed AV delay both affect the primary issue of AV coordination and timing. Ventricular lead positions in the RV outflow tract (RVOT) result in an aberrant activation pattern of myocardial contraction, thereby reducing the pumping efficiency of ventricular systole. If the lead is located on the septal side of the outflow tract, LV activation patterns may also be adversely affected, leading to a reduced stroke volume.

8. c Contraction of the atria during ventricular systole, hence against a closed tricuspid valve, results in transmission of a large pressure wave backwards into the great vessels of the neck, resulting in visible Cannon A-waves. The frequency and relationship of Cannon A-waves and the ventricular rate will depend upon the degree of AV dissociation. An S_3, pulsus paradoxus and systolic ejection murmur may be present, but are not the result of AV dissociation. The fourth heart sound (S_4) is absent with the loss of AV synchrony.

9. b In the presence of chronic atrial fibrillation, revision of the pacing system will have no impact on the return of coordinated AV activity. Answer 'e' is also correct, provided the dual-chamber device is capable of mode switching (the pacemaker automatically reprograms to a mode that is incapable of tracking the atrial rhythm if it classifies the current atrial rhythm as pathologic). When the pacemaker recognizes the atrial rhythm as being physiologic, the pacemaker reprograms back to the previously programmed mode.

10. d While answer 'a' might have initial appeal, the RA pressure falls towards baseline at least two complexes prior to the termination of ventricular pacing. This phenomenon probably represents the loss of (retrograde) VA conduction prior to the onset of sinus rhythm, when the pressure waveform changes to a normal A- and V-wave configuration with correspondingly normal X- and Y-descents. The exaggerated RA pressures during single-chamber ventricular pacing represent Cannon A-waves. There is no reason to suspect a dampened pressure recording.

11. a The irregularly irregular QRS is atrial fibrillation. The LA and RA tracings reveal both small C-waves and large V-waves, consistent with either mitral regurgitation or decreased LA compliance. With close examination, the C-wave is shown to occur after the initiation of the QRS complex, is nearly superimposed on the large V-waves and is reflected in both the RA and LA pressure waveforms. Mechanistically, the C-wave is an interruption in the X-descent that occurs as a result of cardiac motion from early ventricular systole that is transmitted to the atrial chamber by subtle movements in the base of the atria at the atrioventricular plane. Atrial fibrillation does not generate coordinated atrial systolic activity to produce measurable A-waves during hemodynamic recording, and the Y-descent nearly always predominates (see Figure 12.5).

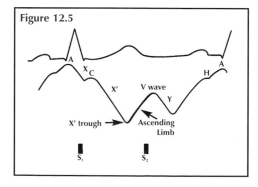

Figure 12.5

12. a In the absence of coordinated atrial activity, no A-wave is generated, therefore no S_4 is produced.

13. d When mitral regurgitation occurs as a result of ischemia, it is generally due to a wall motion abnormality in the endocardium underlying either the anterolateral or posteromedial papillary muscle. This results in a failure of coaptation and eccentric mitral regurgitation. Because both the diagonal and obtuse marginal branches supply the lateral wall, it is uncommon that an infarction in either coronary (alone) will result in enough of a wall motion abnormality to affect the anterolateral papillary muscle. In contrast, the posteromedial papillary muscle, attached to myocardium supplied only by the posterior descending coronary artery, is much more likely to be affected by a single-territory myocardial infarction, resulting in ischemic mitral regurgitation

14. b The presence of V-waves in recorded LA pressures is a sensitive, but not specific, finding of mitral regurgitation.

In RA pressure tracings, the A-wave is generally higher than the V-wave. The opposite is true for the LA, where the pressure waveforms are always more distinct than the PCW waveforms. In PCW pressure tracings, the lower-pressure atrial contraction A-wave amplitude is often attenuated by the pulse-wave transmission through the pulmonary circuit to the distal port of the Swan-Ganz catheter.

The V-wave in a PCW tracing is normally larger than the A-wave. A giant V-wave is defined as a peak pressure twice that of the mean PCW, classically caused by severe mitral regurgitation.

Chapter 13

Left and Right Ventricular Failure

A 53-year-old man develops mild and vague chest discomfort, not alleviated by deep breathing or changing position. He denies past illnesses and takes no medications. Over the past 2 days he developed a dry cough without fever or chills. He had shortness of breath the previous night. Examination reveals bilateral rales, 4 cm of jugular venous distention, a summation gallop and a systolic heart murmur. An electrocardiogram (ECG) showed non-specific ST- and T-wave abnormalities. Cardiac catheterization was performed. Simultaneous pulmonary capillary wedge (PCW) and left ventricular (LV) pressures were recorded (Figure 13.1).

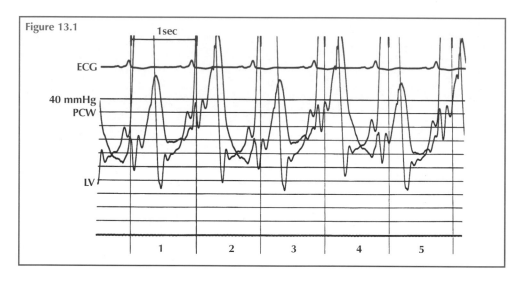

Figure 13.1

1. From the hemodynamic tracing on Figure 13.1 and the clinical history, what is the most likely diagnosis?
   a. Mitral stenosis
   b. Aortic stenosis
   c. Pericardial effusion
   d. Acute tricuspid insufficiency
   e. LV failure

2. In this patient, diagnostic coronary angiography is most likely to reveal:
   a. Angiographically normal arteries
   b. Severe (≥70% diameter stenoses) of the right coronary artery (RCA) only
   c. Mild three-vessel atherosclerosis
   d. Severe (≥70% diameter stenoses) three-vessel atherosclerosis
   e. Anomalous circumflex coronary artery

3. Which of the following waveforms on Figure 13.2 is most commonly associated with valvular incompetence?
   a. A
   b. B
   c. C
   d. D
   e. E

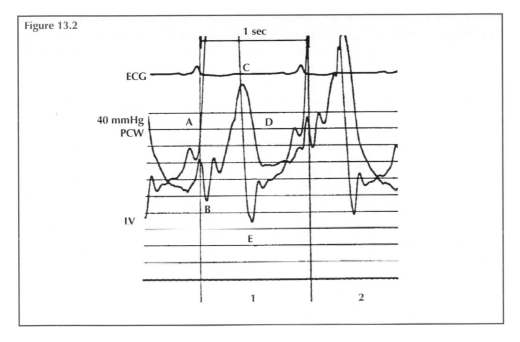

Figure 13.2

4. The hemodynamic tracing on Figure 13.3, obtained 3 days after hospital admission for congestive heart failure (CHF), is most likely to be associated with which of the following?
   a. Removal of 500 mL pericardial fluid
   b. Aggressive treatment with diuretics and afterload reducing agents
   c. Aortic valve replacement
   d. Mitral valve replacement
   e. Insertion of an intra-aortic balloon pump

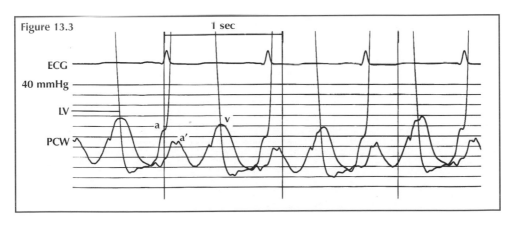

Figure 13.3

A 45-year-old man is referred for rescue balloon angioplasty after an acute inferior myocardial infarction and failed thrombolytic therapy. Prior to the coronary intervention, right heart catheterization reveals the hemodynamic tracings shown in Figures 13.4 and 13.5.

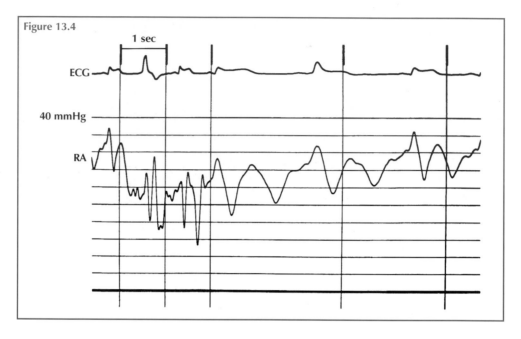

Figure 13.4

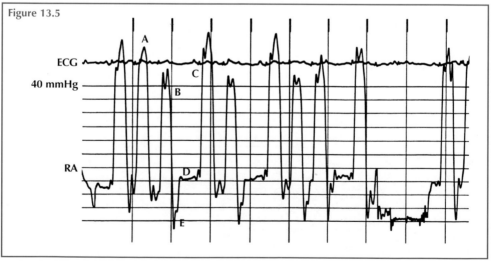

Figure 13.5

5. **Which finding, seen in the right atrial (RA) tracing in Figure 13.4, is least consistent with right ventricular (RV) infarction?**
   a. Elevated mean RA pressure
   b. Large A-wave
   c. Steep Y-descent
   d. Prominent V-wave
   e. M-pattern

6. **Which portion of the RV waveform on Figure 13.5 reflects decreased RV compliance as a result of depressed RV systolic performance and impaired relaxation?**
   a. A
   b. B
   c. C
   d. D
   e. E

7. **Based on Figures 13.4 and 13.5, diagnostic angiography is most likely to demonstrate which of the following?**
   a. Occlusion of the proximal RCA
   b. Occlusion of the mid-RCA
   c. Occlusion of the distal RCA
   d. Occlusion of the posterior descending coronary artery
   e. Occlusion of the circumflex coronary artery

8. **Figure 13.6 demonstrates simultaneous RV and LV recordings before and after percutaneous coronary intervention. Findings indicative of successful reperfusion of the occluded infarct-related artery include all of the following, except:**
    a. Reduction of end-diastolic pressure
    b. Rapid upstroke of RV systolic pressure
    c. Rapid RV relaxation
    d. Persistent matching of the diastolic pressures
    e. Bifid RV systolic waveform

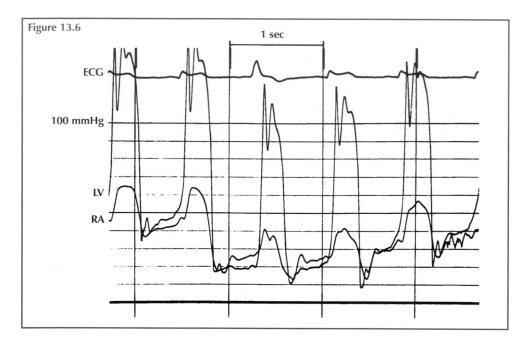

Figure 13.6

Answers

1. **e** Hemodynamic tracings on Figure 13.1 demonstrate several findings. Both the LV end-diastolic pressure (LVEDP) and PCW pressures are elevated. Large V-waves in the PCW tracing also show pressure alternans. These findings are consistent with LV dysfunction and volume overload with or without mitral regurgitation. In this setting, LV failure may be due to several etiologies. The large V-waves suggest mitral regurgitation, which may be due to distortion of the mitral annulus as a result of LV dilation, ischemia of the papillary muscle(s) or mechanical disruption of the valve or substructures due to organic and functional abnormalities (i.e. mitral valve prolapse or chordal rupture).

   Acute mitral insufficiencies resulting from subvalvular chordae rupture are associated with large V-waves with minimal elevations of either LVEDP or mean PCW pressure in the early stages. Mitral stenosis is expected to cause a diastolic LV–PCW gradient, which is not seen on this tracing. Pericardial effusion with tamponade produces diastolic equalization of pressures with a characteristic 'dip and plateau' of the LV diastolic waveform. The LV tracing in Figure 13.1 exhibits rapidly upsloping diastolic pressures (no plateau), consistent with volume overload, and not pericardial constriction or constraint. The diagnosis of aortic stenosis requires both LV and aortic pressures.

2. **d** The most common cause of LV dysfunction in the United States is myocardial ischemia and infarction. Severe LV dysfunction of non-ischemic cardiomyopathy is associated with coronary angiography revealing normal or minimally diseased coronary arteries. An anomalous circumflex coronary artery with coronary artery disease (CAD) may result in myocardial ischemia and infarction, but typically does not produce profound LV dysfunction. Similarly, severe stenosis of the RCA resulting in inferior ischemia may produce acute mitral insufficiency due to papillary muscle dysfunction (with large V waves in the PCW tracing), but is unlikely to result in marked elevations of LVEDP with true RV infarction.

3. **c** This simultaneous PCW and LV tracing exhibits large V-waves that follow LV systole and would be consistent with mitral valve incompetence.

4. **b** Figure 13.3 documents normal LV and PCW pressure waveforms. LV dysfunction resulting from myocardial ischemia may recover following appropriate treatment for excess afterload and preload, as well as improvement in myocardial blood flow. Aggressive treatment with diuretics and afterload reducing agents, such as ACE inhibitors, can be expected to restore normal hemodynamics, particularly in the setting of cardiomyopathy with severe LV dysfunction. The insertion of an intra-aortic balloon pump results in decreased LVED and PCW pressure, but usually will not fully return the LVEDP to normal. This tracing is not consistent with either pericardial effusion with tamponade (filling pressures are normal), or mitral stenosis (no LV–PCW pressure gradient across the mitral valve).

In symptomatic patients with left heart failure, both left and right heart-filling pressures are usually elevated. However, they may be surprisingly normal at rest, as seen in patients with mild systolic dysfunction or after treatment with diuretics or vasodilators. In general, increases in both LV and RV filling pressures are easily induced with physical exercise, explaining why patients may have exertional symptoms only. In the catheterization laboratory, RV decompensation can be elicited with either supine bicycle exercise or arm ergometry. After a few minutes of exercise, PCW pressures can rise up to 30–40 mmHg, and RA pressures can easily reach 15–20 mmHg, demonstrating the loss of LV (and possibly RV) contractile reserve.

Hemodynamically, a slowing of the LV pressure upstroke and downstroke can give a triangular appearance to the LV waveform (as opposed to the almost square or trapezoidal appearance of the normal waveform), often superimposed on elevated diastolic pressures. This effect can be mathematically described by reductions in both the rate of rise ($+dP/dt$) and fall ($-dP/dt$) in LV pressures during systole.

In mild CHF, the cardiac index may be normal or only slightly reduced, whereas in more severe cases the cardiac output is commonly reduced more significantly. A cardiac index (CI) of 1.5 L/min/m^2 or less indicates an advanced depression of cardiac performance and a poor prognosis.

In LV dysfunction, both systemic and pulmonary vascular resistances (SVR and PVR) are often elevated. Because cardiac output is reduced, modest increases in SVR do not result in elevation of the systemic blood pressure (BP), but rather tend to preserve the BP at a normal or only slightly reduced level.

The reduction of SVR and PVR following administration of intravenous vasodilators can result in a striking increase in cardiac output with a simultaneous reduction in both LV and RV filling pressures. A favorable result following nitroprusside challenge in the catheterization lab predicts that the long-term response to oral vasodilators may be positive. Intravenous inotropes, such as dobutamine, can also exhibit the same effect. It is on this hemodynamic basis that many patients with extremely advanced CHF benefit from prolonged (72 h or greater) infusions of these agents.

5. c RV infarction produces both systolic and diastolic dysfunction. As a result of RV functional impairment, RA pressures are increased. The hemodynamic waveforms may resemble those of constrictive physiology. A blunted RA Y-descent is indicative of diastolic resistance to RV filling. As a result of increased filling pressures, the force of RA systole is exaggerated, producing a rapid upstroke and increased amplitude of the A-wave. Depending on the site of RCA occlusion, RA relaxation may be enhanced or impaired. Enhanced relaxation is reflected by a steep X-descent (W- or M-pattern, see Figure 13.7). If the RA is also ischemic (as may be the case with a very proximal RCA occlusion), atrial function may be depressed, which manifests as an elevated mean RA pressure with depressed A-wave and less striking X-descent (M-pattern). Prominent V-waves are produced by passive atrial filling or, when exaggerated, are due to tricuspid regurgitation.

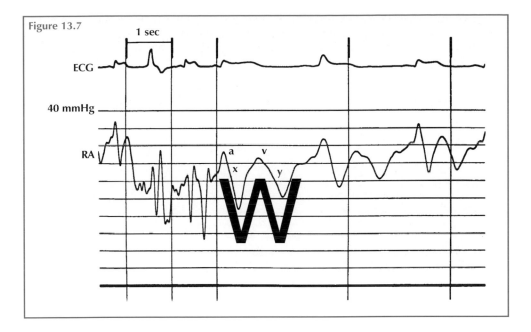

Figure 13.7

6. **d** Acute ischemia of the RV free wall impedes both systolic and diastolic RV function. Hemodynamic tracings may reveal a slow RV upstroke, decreased peak RV pressure and/or delayed relaxation. Severe RV diastolic dysfunction produces a dilated and stiff RV (decreased compliance), which is reflected in severely increased filling pressures resulting from increased impedance to inflow. At some point, pericardial constraint becomes physiologically important, affecting RV filling pressures and limiting RV end-diastolic volume. The resistance to diastolic filling, for either pericardial restraint or RV infarction, is manifest in the RV waveform as a rapid rise in diastolic pressure to an elevated plateau (the flat portion of the characteristic 'dip and plateau'), as shown in this case example. The comparatively blunted Y-descent (compared to the X-descent, see Figure 13.7) can be used to distinguish RV infarction from the predominant and sharp Y-descent seen in isolated pericardial constriction.

Patients with RV infarction often present with striking abnormalities of right heart hemodynamics. In its most severe form, the syndrome of predominant RV infarction is characterized by right heart failure, with clear lung fields and hypotension. Clinically, RV infarction patients are preload dependent, often requiring significant fluid resuscitation in the early stages of therapy.

Hemodynamic evaluation in RV infarction patients typically reveals disproportionate elevation of right heart filling pressure, equalization of right and left-sided diastolic pressures and low cardiac output despite LV function. Simultaneous RV and LV hemodynamic patterns in RV infarct patients often demonstrate constrictive or restrictive physiology, resulting from pericardial constraint applied to the dilating RV.

RV systolic dysfunction, manifest in the RV waveform by a slow upstroke, diminished peak pressures and delayed relaxation, reduces transpulmonary flow and results in diminished LV preload and decreased cardiac output despite preserved LV contractility.

Acute RV dilatation and elevated RV pressures shift the interventricular septum towards the volume-deprived LV, thereby impairing LV compliance and further limiting LV diastolic filling. Abrupt RV dilatation with the non-compliant pericardium leads to elevated intrapericardial pressures due to pericardial constraint, impairing both RV and LV compliance and filling, further intensifying the adverse effects of diastolic ventricular interactions. Pericardial constraint further contributes to the progressive pandiastolic impedance of RV filling, reflected hemodynamically by a blunted RA Y-descent, RV 'dip and plateau' pattern and elevated and equalized RV/LV diastolic filling pressures.

7. **b** Inspection of the RV and RA waveforms reveals an augmented A-wave and a blunted or delayed Y-descent indicating decreased RV compliance and augmented atrial contractility. These findings are consistent with infarction that spares the RA. In contrast, RA infarction results in decreased atrial systolic function (diminished A-wave) and delayed X-descent (the M-pattern). Occlusion of the mid-RCA is most likely to cause infarction of only the RV, sparing the RA. A proximal RCA occlusion can result in atrial ischemia or infarction, and severe hypotension. Conversely, occlusion of the distal RCA or posterior descending artery (PDA) is unlikely to affect RV systolic function, and more likely to result in ischemia of the inferior segment of the LV. Distal branches of the circumflex coronary artery rarely supply significant RV branches.

8. **d** Successful reperfusion of an occluded RCA is expected to resolve the hemodynamic effects of severe RV ischemia, depending upon the amount of irreversible tissue injury and cellular death ('stunning' vs. infarction). Therefore, waveform analysis is expected to reveal resolution of both systolic and diastolic dysfunction.

Restoration of systolic performance is reflected by a rapid upstroke of RV systolic pressure and increased peak RV systolic pressure. Improved diastolic function manifests with rapid ventricular filling and increased RV compliance. This produces a reduction in end-diastolic pressure and resolution of the 'dip and plateau' contour. The relative matching of RV and LV diastolic pressures is a non-specific finding that may indicate persistent mild diastolic dysfunction, volume overload and/or pericardial constraint following significant RV ischemic dilation.

A bifid systolic RV waveform may be found during RV infarction as a result of unopposed LV-septal pressure generation. Paradoxical early systolic bulging into the RV cavity produces the early peak, whereas maximal LV-septal shortening and peak systolic pressure generation produce the second peak.

Chapter 14
Pulmonary Hypertension

A 61-year-old woman presented to the emergency room complaining of intermittent crushing chest pain with severe dyspnea at rest. She was referred for immediate cardiac catheterization and coronary angiography. During right heart cardiac catheterization she developed her typical recurrent chest pain and dyspnea, both of which spontaneously resolved in minutes. The hemodynamic responses are shown on Figure 14.1 (note different pressure scale).

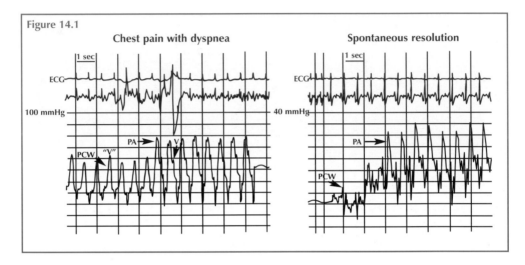

Figure 14.1

1. What is the most likely etiology of this patient's severe, but reversible, pulmonary hypertension?
   a. Pulmonary embolism
   b. Acute coronary syndrome with papillary muscle dysfunction
   c. Mitral stenosis
   d. Primary pulmonary hypertension
   e. Pulmonic valve stenosis

For Questions 2–5, choose the most likely patient and associated hemodynamic findings for each cause of pulmonary hypertension.

| Patient | CO (L/min) | Pressure (mmHg) | | | | PVR (Wood units) |
		Mean PA	Mean PCW	Mean RA	LVED	
1	3.5	40	10	10	8	8.5
2	3.5	70	10	15	10	17.1
3	3.5	60	20	20	20	11.4
4	3.5	60	30	20	10	8.5

CO: cardiac output; LVED: left ventricular end-diastolic; PA: pulmonary artery;
PCW: pulmonary capillary wedge; PVR: pulmonary vascular resistance; RA: right atrial.

2. **Primary pulmonary hypertension:**
    a. 1
    b. 2
    c. 3
    d. 4

3. **Dilated cardiomyopathy:**
    a. 1
    b. 2
    c. 3
    d. 4

4. **Acute (new onset) pulmonary embolus:**
    a. 1
    b. 2
    c. 3
    d. 4

5. **Mitral stenosis:**
    a. 1
    b. 2
    c. 3
    d. 4

6. **How is PVR calculated?**
    a. (PA systolic PA diastolic) / PA systolic
    b. (PA systolic - PA diastolic) / PA diastolic
    c. (PA mean - PCW mean) / CO
    d. (PA mean + PCW mean) / Cardiac index
    e. PA systolic / PCW mean

7. **Typically, which of the following conditions is not associated with right ventricular (RV) pressure overload?**
    a. Severe mitral stenosis
    b. Chronic thromboembolic disease
    c. Chronic obstructive pulmonary disease (COPD)
    d. Severe tricuspid regurgitation
    e. Systemic sclerosis

8. **All of the following drugs have been shown to reduce PVR in primary pulmonary hypertension except:**
    a. Hydralazine
    b. Nifedipine
    c. Prostacyclin
    d. Nitric oxide
    e. Metoprolol

Answers

1. **b** During an episode of spontaneous myocardial ischemia, this patient developed sudden and extreme pulmonary hypertension. The key finding is the presence of very large V-waves within the PCW pressure tracing, suggesting acute mitral valve regurgitation as an etiology. Nitroglycerin reduces preload very effectively thereby reducing RV filling pressures. Recurrent (or multiple) pulmonary embolism can be associated with large V-waves in the wedge position. Mitral stenosis is not associated with this degree of variability of the pulmonary artery (PA) pressures, except during active exercise. Primary pulmonary hypertension is not spontaneously (or rapidly) reversible. Pulmonic valve stenosis is associated with an RV–PA pressure gradient, not demonstrated in this example.

2. **b** Patients with primary pulmonary hypertension typically show markedly elevated PA pressures and pulmonary vascular resistance (PVR), with normal LV pressures. Cardiac output may be reduced, due to decreased venous return and, ultimately, RV failure.

Pulmonary arterial hypertension may be caused by hypoxic pulmonary vasoconstriction (e.g. COPD), destruction of normal lung parenchyma (e.g. interstitial lung disease), obliterative pulmonary vascular disease (e.g. chronic pulmonary emboli, systemic sclerosis), pulmonary venous hypertension (e.g. mitral valve disease or LV dysfunction), chronic volume overload (e.g. atrial septal defect) or it may be idiopathic (e.g. primary pulmonary hypertension). The RV hypertrophies in order to preserve RV systolic function. As PA pressures and resistance rise, the RV is eventually unable to compensate and begins to dilate, resulting in worsening RV function and, ultimately, cor pulmonale.

3. **c** This patient has classic features of biventricular dysfunction, with elevated left and right-sided filling pressures, pulmonary venous hypertension and reduced cardiac output.

4. **a** Although pulmonary hypertension is a hallmark of chronic pulmonary embolism, a previously healthy RV is only capable of generating a mean PA pressure of approximately 40 mmHg before onset of hemodynamic collapse. Cardiac output and LVEDP are low, as a result of under-filling of the LV due to RV failure.

5. **d** In the case of mitral stenosis, high LA pressure leads to pulmonary venous hypertension, and, eventually, pulmonary arterial hypertension. Pulmonary pressure is frequently elevated out-of-proportion to LA pressure, while the LV is spared (normal LV end-diastolic pressures).

6. **c** The normal pulmonary vascular bed offers less than 10% of the resistance to flow compared to the systemic bed. PVR is generally quantified as the ratio of pressure drop to mean flow (Q, measured in L/min). The ratio is commonly multiplied by 79.9 (rounded to 80 for simplification) for metric conversion (dynes/s/cm^{-5}). Alternatively, this conversion can be avoided, leaving the resistance in units of mmHg/L/min, which are often referred to as hybrid units, peripheral resistance units (PRU) or Wood units (named after the English cardiologist Paul Wood).

The calculated PVR in a normal adult is 67 ± 23 dynes/s/cm^{-5}, or 1 Wood unit. Pulmonary hypertension is believed to be irreversible if the calculated resistance reaches 4 Wood units. Dividing DP by the cardiac index provides the commonly reported pulmonary vascular resistance index (PVRI).

7. **d** Tricuspid regurgitation causes RV failure due to chronic volume overload – pulmonary arterial pressure is usually normal or minimally elevated ('low-pressure' volume overload). All other choices are associated with RV pressure overload states.

8. **e** Hydralazine, nifedipine, prostacyclin and nitric oxide are all known to reduce PA pressure and PVR. These drugs share marked vasodilatory properties. There is currently no proven role for the use of β-adrenoreceptor blocking agents in the treatment of primary pulmonary hypertension.

Once severe pulmonary hypertension has developed, the prognosis is poor, regardless of the cause. Often, clinical status may improve with treatment of the underlying etiology (i.e. mitral valve replacement or chronic oxygen therapy). Medical therapy for pulmonary hypertension is often directed at reducing pulmonary vascular resistance with vasodilators. Symptoms of right-sided heart failure may be relieved with diuretics. Single or bilateral lung transplantation is an additional therapeutic option for patients with intrinsic lung disease.

Chapter 15
Intra-aortic Balloon Pumping

A 52-year-old man presents to the emergency department with an acute anterior myocardial infarction and cardiogenic shock. In addition to infusing vasopressor agents, an intra-aortic balloon pump (IABP) is inserted for hemodynamic support. The hemodynamic pressure tracings are shown on Figure 15.1.

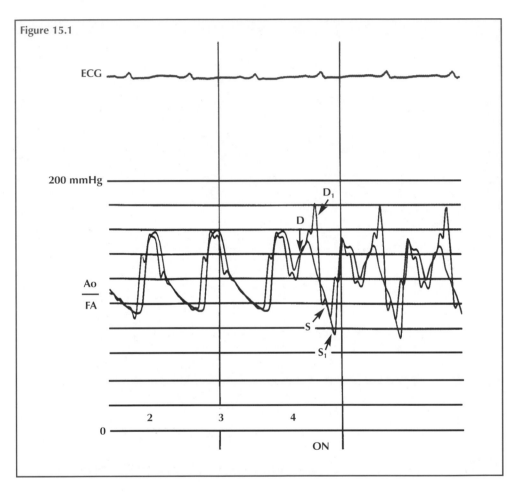

Figure 15.1

1. **Which of the following is not an indication for IABP placement?**
   a. Cardiogenic shock in a patient awaiting heart transplant
   b. Medically refractory unstable angina
   c. Cardiac tamponade
   d. High-risk percutaneous transluminal coronary angioplasty (PTCA)
   e. Malignant arrhythmia due to ongoing ischemia

2. Which of the following is not a contraindication of IABP placement?
    a. Severe aortic regurgitation
    b. Concomitant use of thrombolytic therapy
    c. Severe bilateral atherosclerotic peripheral vascular disease
    d. Abdominal aortic aneurysm
    e. Suspected aortic dissection

3. Which of the following is not a physiologic benefit of IABP?
    a. Increased coronary perfusion pressure
    b. Increased cardiac output
    c. Decreased myocardial oxygen demand
    d. Increased myocardial contractility
    e. Decreased left ventricular (LV) afterload

Questions 4–6 refer to the aortic pressure tracing on Figure 15.2.

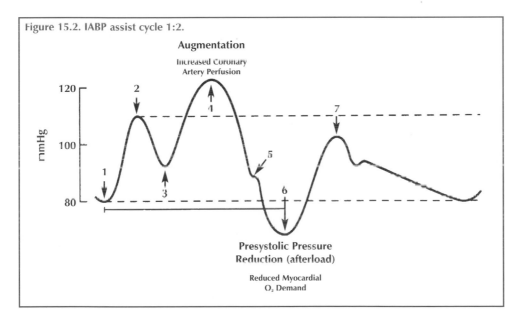

Figure 15.2. IABP assist cycle 1:2.

4. At which point does balloon inflation occur?
    a. 1
    b. 2
    c. 3
    d. 4
    e. 6

5. **Which point indicates aortic systolic pressure during IABP?**
   a. 1
   b. 2
   c. 3
   d. 4
   e. 7

6. **Which point indicates diastolic pressure augmentation?**
   a. 1
   b. 2
   c. 3
   d. 4
   e. 6

7. **What is the most common complication of IABP placement?**
   a. Hemolysis
   b. Balloon rupture
   c. Sepsis
   d. Limb ischemia
   e. Arterial dissection

Answers

1. **c** The IABP is an adjunctive and established mechanical support to pharmacological treatment of the failing heart after myocardial infarction, unstable angina and cardiac surgery. Although it is much less efficient at supporting the systemic circulation than some more recently introduced devices (LV or RV assist devices, percutaneous cardiopulmonary bypass support, etc.), the IABP remains the most commonly used mechanical support device because of its simplicity, ease of insertion and long clinical track record.

IABP insertion and use provide for a more favorable myocardial oxygen supply/demand balance than pharmacologic support alone. During balloon deflation, afterload is reduced (thereby reducing myocardial oxygen requirements), and during balloon inflation, diastolic pressure is augmented (improving myocardial oxygen supply). The overall net hemodynamic effects are an increased stroke volume, cardiac output and coronary perfusion. Human studies have demonstrated that, in patients with acute coronary occlusion, the IABP-augmented diastolic perfusion pressure results in a redistribution of coronary blood flow towards ischemic areas of the myocardium.

Routine IABP insertion prior to cardiac surgery is usually reserved for patients with angina refractory to medical therapy, severe left main stenosis or those with very low cardiac output. In this population, IABP support has been shown to reduce hospital mortality and shorten the course of intensive care.

Indications for IABP
Refractory unstable angina
Cardiogenic shock
Postoperative hemodynamic compromise
Acute myocardial infarction with mechanical impairment as a result of mitral regurgitation or ventricular septal defect
Intractable ventricular tachycardia as a result of myocardial ischemia
Patients with left main coronary artery (LMCA) stenosis or severe 3-vessel disease undergoing anesthesia for cardiac surgery
High risk PTCA
Maintenance of vessel patency after PTCA of a total occlusion

The hemodynamic derangements of cardiac tamponade result from inadequate cardiac filling, and are not improved with either afterload reduction or diastolic pressure augmentation that is achieved with effective IABP support.

2. **b** Although the risk of bleeding from the arteriotomy site is increased in this setting, the use of thrombolytic therapy is not a contraindication of IABP.

Contraindications for IABP placement
Anatomic abnormality of femoral-iliac artery
Iliac or aortic atherosclerotic disease impairing blood flow run-off
Moderate or severe aortic valve regurgitation
Aortic dissection or aneurysm
Patent ductus (counterpulsation may augment the abnormal pathway from aortic to pulmonary artery)
Bypass grafting to femoral arteries or aorta
Bleeding diathesis
Sepsis

3. **d** IABP increases myocardial oxygen supply (e.g. coronary perfusion pressure), decreases myocardial oxygen demand, increases cardiac output and decreases LV afterload. While overall cardiac performance is improved, there is no direct positive inotropic effect.

4. **c** Balloon inflation is timed to begin immediately after closure of the aortic valve, indicated by the dicrotic notch.

5. **e** The systolic pressure waveform immediately following balloon deflation reflects the effect of a reduction in afterload on (intrinsic) systolic pressure.

6. **d**

7. **d** While all the complications listed are associated with IABP placement, limb ischemia occurs most frequently. Early ischemia usually results from physical obstruction to arterial flow by the large introducer sheath. Late ischemia is usually the result of thrombus accumulation around the sheath. Sepsis is a contraindication to IABP placement, but not usually a complication of the procedure.

   Most complications of IABP placement related to local vascular insufficiency can be resolved without permanent sequelae. Whereas the rate of significant IABP-related complications is approximately 10%, permanent morbidity is <5% and IABP-related mortality is <1%. Complications are more frequent in women and diabetic or hypertensive patients, but there is no convincing evidence to relate this to the duration of counterpulsation.

Chapter 16
Coronary Hemodynamics

A 52-year-old man with an atypical chest pain syndrome, hiatal hernia and hypertension presents for cardiac catheterization. Coronary angiography is performed. Two intermediately severe coronary stenoses are noted.

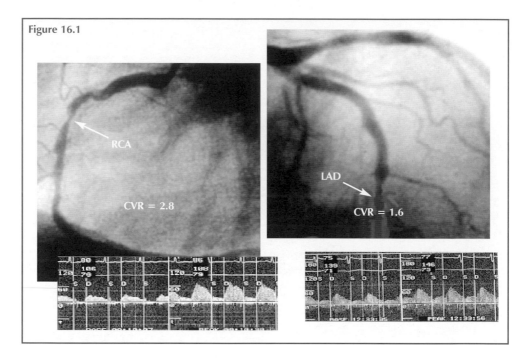

Figure 16.1

1. **Based on the coronary flow velocity reserve (CVR) for each artery shown in Figure 16.1, which of the following statements is correct?**
   a. CVR for lesions >70% cannot exceed 2.5
   b. CVR for lesions <40% is always >2.5
   c. Relative CVR (rCVR) is 0.57
   d. rCVR is 0.88
   e. The right coronary artery (RCA) should be dilated

A 72-year-old woman has a severe circumflex coronary artery stenosis. The left anterior descending artery is normal. The hemodynamics of fractional flow reserve (FFR), absolute and relative CVR are shown in Figure 16.2.

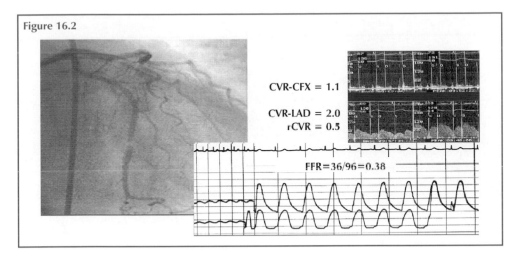

Figure 16.2

CVR-CFX = 1.1

CVR-LAD = 2.0
rCVR = 0.5

FFR=36/96=0.38

2. Based on these data, which of the following statements is true?
   a. CVR of the circumflex artery is abnormal due to microvascular disease
   b. CVR of the left anterior descending artery is abnormal
   c. FFR is abnormal due to microvascular disease
   d. CVR of <2.0 is associated with microvascular disease
   e. rCVR of >0.8 does not exclude microvascular disease

3. After coronary angioplasty of the circumflex artery, CVR is improved from 1.1 to 1.5 (Figure 16.3). Which of the following does not contribute to this phenomenon?
   a. Residual lumen narrowing
   b. Diffuse disease
   c. Normalization of the microcirculation
   d. Resetting of basal coronary flow
   e. Microvascular stunning

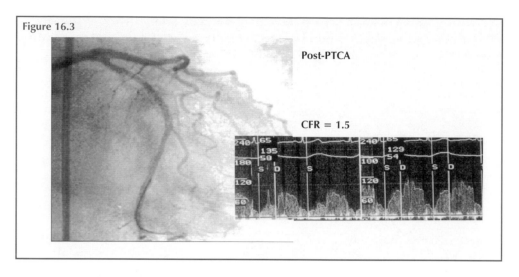

Figure 16.3

Post-PTCA

CFR = 1.5

4. Figure 16.4 shows the CVR and FFR data obtained after stent placement. Which of the following is the most appropriate next step?
   a. Post-dilate with same size balloon, but at higher pressures
   b. Intravascular (coronary) ultrasound (IVUS)
   c. Post-dilate with a larger balloon, because CVR of the circumflex is only 2.0
   d. No further treatment is indicated
   e. Additional stenting is needed

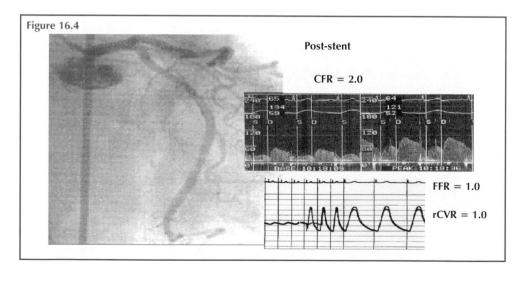

Figure 16.4

Post-stent

CFR = 2.0

FFR = 1.0

rCVR = 1.0

A 58-year-old man with angina and positive stress echocardiography, suggesting inferior ischemia, has serial RCA stenoses of intermediate severity in each of two projections. FFR data obtained beyond the more distal of the two stenoses are shown on Figure 16.5.

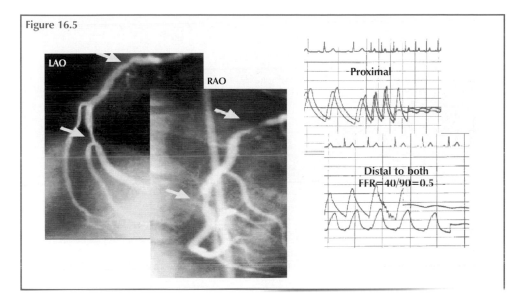

Figure 16.5

5.   Which of the following is indicated by these data?
   a. Only the proximal lesion is severe
   b. Only the distal lesion is severe
   c. Neither lesion is severe
   d. Cannot determine individual lesion severity with available data
   e. An FFR of 0.5 represents the measurement artifact

6. Following coronary angioplasty of only the proximal lesion, the following FFR data (again distal to both stenoses) were recorded (Figure 16.6). What is the clinical implication of this finding?
   a. The proximal lesion is inadequately dilated
   b. The distal lesion is inadequately dilated
   c. The distal lesion should be stented
   d. IVUS is needed
   e. No further intervention is needed

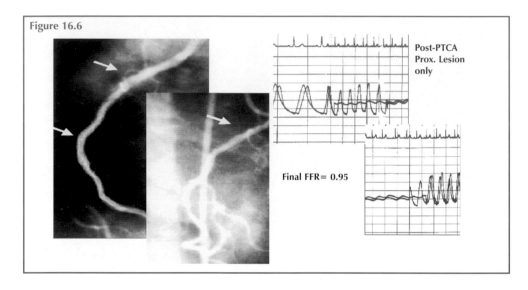

Figure 16.6

Post-PTCA
Prox. Lesion
only

Final FFR= 0.95

A 52-year-old physician has a chest pain syndrome with positive stress perfusion imaging in the anterior wall. FFR data are presented in Figure 16.7.

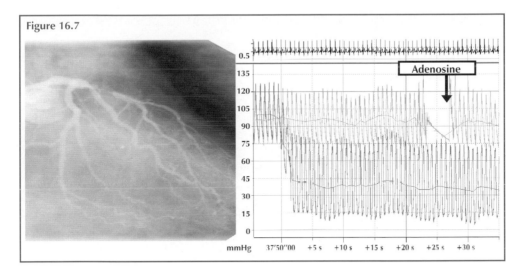

Figure 16.7

7. Regarding Figure 16.7, which of the following statements is the most correct?
   a. A resting gradient of 60 mmHg (P_{aorta} - P_{distal} = 95 - 35 mmHg) is significant; proceed directly with coronary intervention
   b. A resting gradient of 20 mmHg is sufficient to proceed directly with intervention
   c. FFR = 0.65
   d. FFR may be influenced by low flow (i.e. microvascular disease)
   e. Intracoronary adenosine produced a large increase in coronary flow in this coronary artery

After coronary stenting of the proximal left anterior descending (LAD) artery, FFR measurements in the mid- and distal-LAD artery are shown on Figure 16.8. With pressure wire pullback from distal to proximal, continuous pressures are recorded during hyperemia as shown in Figure 16.9.

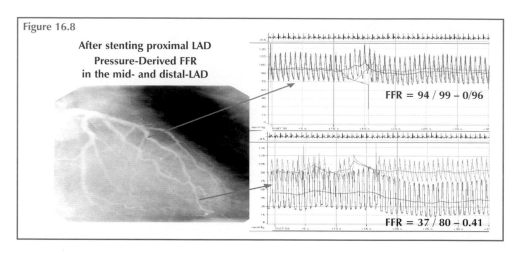

Figure 16.8

After stenting proximal LAD
Pressure-Derived FFR
in the mid- and distal-LAD

FFR = 94 / 99 – 0/96

FFR = 37 / 80 – 0.41

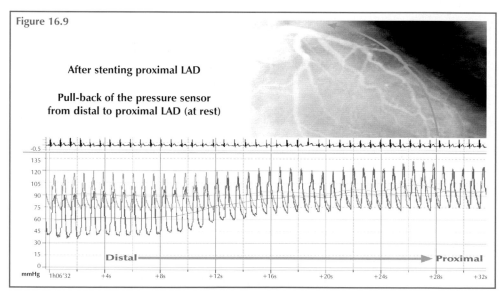

Figure 16.9

After stenting proximal LAD

Pull-back of the pressure sensor
from distal to proximal LAD (at rest)

Distal ⟶ Proximal

8. Based on Figures 16.8 and 16.9, which of the following statements is most correct?
   a. The stent for the primary lesion in the proximal vessel is not well deployed
   b. The distal artery needs additional stenting
   c. The abnormal distal FFR is due to diffuse coronary artery disease
   d. There is no angiographic reason to explain why the distal pressure is lower than the proximal pressure, making artifact very likely
   e. There is guide catheter damping during pullback

A 48-year-old man with hypertension and hyperlipidemia presents feeling weak and dizzy with palpitations. The admission electrocardiogram (ECG) revealed intermittent wide complex tachycardia during these short-lived episodes. Cardiac catheterization revealed only a 50–60% lesion in the proximal left circumflex coronary artery. An intracoronary pressure wire was used to assess the severity of the lesion. On crossing the lesion, a large pressure gradient was found (see Figure 16.10).

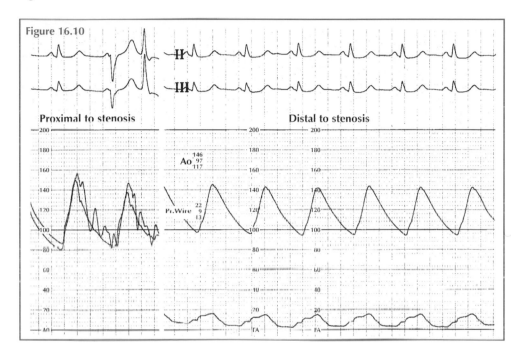

9. On the basis of the resting pressure gradient across the left circumflex lesion (Figure 16.10), which of the following statements is most correct?
   a. The stenosis is angiographically and physiologically non-obstructive to coronary blood flow; no further testing is required
   b. The stenosis is angiographically obstructive, but has no significant physiologic limitation to coronary flow
   c. The stenosis is physiologically obstructive to flow; immediate percutaneous intervention is indicated without further testing
   d. The physiologic significance of the stenosis may be exaggerated by coronary vasospasm; an intracoronary vasodilator (e.g. nitroglycerin) should be administered
   e. A technical problem with the pressure wire has been encountered; an alternative method should be used for ischemic testing

Intracoronary nitroglycerin (200 μg) was given, and the resting pressure gradient across the coronary stenosis was re-measured (Figure 16.11, panel A). Using intracoronary adenosine (24 μg) an FFR measurement was also taken (Figure 16.11, panel B).

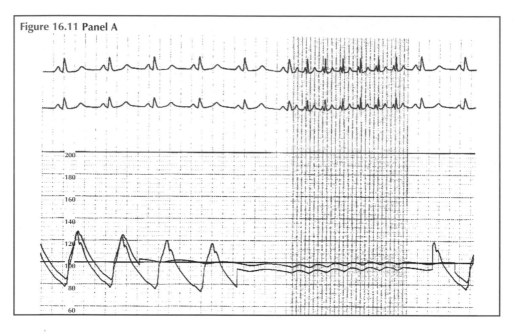

Figure 16.11 Panel A

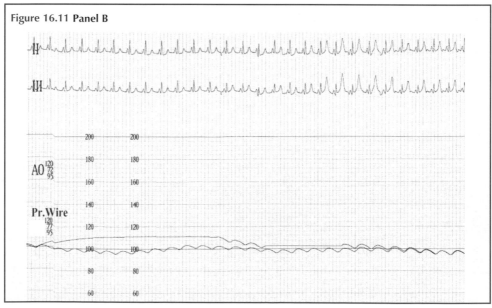

Figure 16.11 Panel B

10. **Based on the tracings on Figure 16.11, which of the following is the most likely diagnostic explanation?**
    a. Spontaneous coronary artery vasospasm
    b. Pressure-wire induced vasospasm
    c. Occluding thrombus is present in the coronary artery
    d. The lesion is physiologically obstructive to flow
    e. A technical problem with the pressure wire has been encountered

11. **Coronary vasospasm is associated with all of following except:**
    a. Rest pain associated with non-specific or no ECG changes
    b. Rest pain associated with transient ST- segment elevation or ventricular dysrhythmias
    c. Rest pain associated with preserved effort tolerance
    d. Angina associated with ST-segment depression during stress testing
    e. Rest pain associated with cyclic recurrence, often early in the morning

12. **Contraindications for ergonovine provocative testing include all of the following except:**
    a. Amenorrhea in pre-menopausal females
    b. Severe hypertension
    c. Severe aortic stenosis
    d. Significant left main coronary artery stenosis
    e. Angina associated with ST-segment elevation during stress testing

13. **All of the following statements regarding ergonovine-induced coronary vasospasm are true except:**
    a. Vasospasm is inducible in 15% of patients with atypical chest pain
    b. Vasospasm is inducible in 15% of patients with symptoms of either exertional or resting angina
    c. Vasospasm can occur in angiographically normal coronary arteries
    d. Vasospasm is inducible in 15% of patients with recorded ST segment elevation during rest angina
    e. Vasospasm commonly occurs in atherosclerotic coronary arteries

14. **Which of the following is the most appropriate initial management recommendation for patients with ventricular tachycardia associated with inducible vasospasm in an angiographically normal coronary artery?**
    a. Referral for electrophysiologic testing
    b. Type I(c) anti-arrhythmic agents
    c. Direct referral for intracoronary device (ICD) implantation
    d. Calcium channel blocking agents, with or without nitrates
    e. β-blocking agents

Answers

1. c The rCVR is the ratio of target vessel CVR to a (normal) reference vessel CVR. Although there is no angiographically normal vessel in this case, the RCA serves as a 'normal' reference since CVR is normal at 2.8. The LAD target vessel CVR is 1.6, yielding an rCVR of 1.6 / 2.8 = 0.57. In this case, the RCA has normal CVR (>2.5) and the patient would not benefit from RCA coronary intervention.

An epicardial stenosis produces an increased resistance to blood flow. In response to decreased flow, the distant microvascular resistance vessels dilate to maintain regional basal flow at a level appropriate for concurrent myocardial oxygen demand. Therefore, the increased capacitance of the vascular bed reduces the potential maximal flow (reserve) available.

The resting post-stenotic epicardial blood flow is unchanged from its normal level until the stenosis becomes very severe (usually >90% narrowed). Resting flow maintains myocardial systolic function, oxidative metabolism and cellular viability. In the presence of a significant stenosis, any further increase in myocardial oxygen demand (or other hyperemic stimuli) will result in reduced post-stenotic hyperemia relative to the coronary flow increase that would occur in the same (or another) myocardial region without a stenosis. A blunted post-stenotic hyperemia (CVR) can be easily identified in the catheterization laboratory measuring Doppler coronary flow in response to a pharmacologic hyperemic stimulus, such as intracoronary adenosine or papaverine or measuring coronary flow velocity.

As a companion to diminished *flow*, a significant stenosis also produces a loss of post-stenotic arterial pressure because of a loss of kinetic energy due to viscous friction, turbulence and flow separation. The reduction of the distal arterial pressure results in a pressure gradient between the aortic and distal coronary pressure. This *pressure* gradient, measured during a similar pharmacologic hyperemic stimulus (i.e. adenosine), is the FFR (fractional flow reserve).

Microvascular disease is defined in the catheterization lab as a CVR of <2.0, in the absence of obstructive macrovascular disease. Microvascular disease impairs the ability of a coronary bed to accommodate increases in coronary blood flow. Microvascular disease will not influence FFR, which is measured as the ratio of distal pressure across a stenosis to aortic pressure during hyperemia.

Relative CVR
A normal absolute CVR indicates a normal 2-component system with a patent epicardial conduit supplying a normal myocardial bed. In the absence of a stenosis, CVR may still be abnormal due to a compromised microvascular circulation (e.g., left ventricular hypertrophy, chronic or acute myocardial ischemia or diabetes mellitus). A low CVR does not indicate which of these two components is abnormal. To confirm coronary lesion significance in this setting, an additional measurement of CVR in an adjacent, normal vessel ($CVR_{reference}$) is used.

$$rCVR = \frac{CVR \text{ (target vessel)}}{CVR \text{ (reference vessel)}}$$

Intermediate angiographic stenoses (40–70% severity) are associated with normal or abnormal coronary blood flow. Physiologic assessments, using either CVR or FFR in this subgroup of angiographically intermediate stenoses, can be clinically important and useful in guiding therapy or predicting long-term outcome following an intervention. The differences between CVR, rCVR and FFR are shown in Figure 16.12.

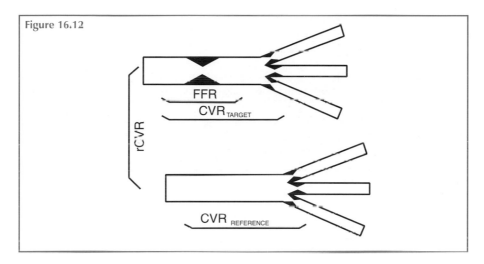

Figure 16.12

FFR was derived by Pijls et al. as a new concept in pressure derived measurement of coronary perfusion. The FFR is the fraction of maximal coronary blood flow that traverses the stenotic vessel as a percentage of blood flow through the same artery in the theoretical absence of stenosis. The FFR reflects the myocardial perfusion rather than merely a stenosis gradient and is differentiated from CVR by being independent of hemodynamic and microcirculatory factors. The ratio of the absolute distal coronary to aortic pressures measured during maximal hyperemia (i.e., when minimal resistance is present across both the epicardial and microvascular beds) yields the FFR.

The normal value for FFR is unequivocally 1 for each patient, coronary artery, myocardial distribution and microcirculatory status. Calculation of an FFR value of <0.75 in patients with stable angina is strongly related to provokable myocardial ischemia using multiple stress testing methods. Therefore, FFR is theoretically a more lesion-specific measurement when compared to absolute CVR or resting trans-stenotic pressure gradients.

Although there is some variance in the literature, widely accepted cut-off values (below which a stenosis is believed to be physiologically obstructing distal coronary flow or flow reserve) are listed below.

	Abnormal	Normal
FFR	<0.75*	1.0
CVR	< 2.0*	>2.0
rCVR	< 0.80*	>0.8

*associated wtih ischemic responses on stress testing or perfusion imaging

2. **d** In this case the circumflex CVR = 1.1 and the FFR = 0.38. When considered together, these measurements suggest that the stenosis itself is responsible for the impairment in hyperemic flow. Although a reduced CVR may be due to microvascular disease, the reduced FFR is independent of microvascular disease.

   The rCVR can be used to characterize the significance of an angiographically intermediate stenosis in the presence of microvascular disease, but alone does not exclude microvascular disease. An rCVR of >0.8 does not exclude microvascular disease, since both the target and reference vessels may be affected by the same microvascular impairment. A CVR in the LAD of 2.0 is within the accepted normal range (CVR < 2.0). A CVR of <2.0 suggests microvascular impairment, but may also represent a physiologically significant (flow-limiting) coronary stenosis.

3. **c** An impaired CVR following balloon angioplasty is often due to residual material in the lumen (which is unappreciated by angiography) that remains physiologically limiting to flow. Diffuse coronary disease may also impair coronary flow despite an adequate post-percutaneous transluminal coronary angioplasty (PTCA) lumen. Resetting of basal flow may occur, especially in the first minutes after angioplasty, as noted in this patient showing a high basal flow velocity of 60 cm/s. The increase in basal flow will mathematically reduce the calculated CVR. Microvascular stunning due to particulate matter embolization has also been suggested as a cause of transiently impaired CVR after PTCA.

4. **d** Following stenting, the target vessel CVR is equal to that of the unobstructed reference vessel, as indicated by the rCVR of 1. Additionally, the FFR is also normal (FFR = 1.0), indicating that no pressure is lost across the stent. Based on this information, no further intervention is indicated.

   IVUS is not necessary, since FFR and CVR have been normalized. Hannekamp et al., have demonstrated that an FFR of >0.94 correlates to IVUS imaging showing full stent deployment in over 91% of cases. Additional stenting is not required because measured coronary physiology is now normal.

5. **d** Serial coronary stenoses cannot be individually assessed using FFR or CVR values, since flow impairment due to the proximal lesion may limit the hyperemia across the more distal lesion. Based on the available data, the distal FFR of 0.5 indicates that both lesions together are physiologically significant. Serial dilatation of the proximal and the distal lesion (or vice versa, at the operator's discretion) can be performed with sequential assessments of FFR after each intervention.

   There is no reason to suggest that an FFR of 0.50 is an artifact based on the quality of the wave form.

6. **e** Based on the FFR of 0.95 after dilatation of only the proximal lesion, there is no need to further dilate either the proximal or distal lesion. Stenting is probably not necessary, since clinical outcomes of FFR-guided angioplasty indicate that for a post-PTCA FFR of >0.90, restenosis rates are <15% at 2 years (Bech GJ, De Bruyne B, Pijls NH et al. Fractional flow reserve to determine the appropriateness of angioplasty in moderate coronary stenosis: a randomized trial. Circulation 2001;103:2928–34).

7. **a** In this severe left anterior descending lesion, a resting gradient of 60 mmHg is sufficient to proceed directly with intervention (a resting ratio of distal artery pressure to proximal aortic pressure of 35/95 mmHg exceeds the FFR limit of ischemia of <0.75). A resting gradient of 20 mmHg is not sufficient to justify proceeding directly with intervention. FFR is not needed for this critical lesion, based on the clinical presentation and the resting pressure ratio (Pd/Pa) across the stenosis. After adenosine injection, the FFR remains essentially unchanged (FFR = 35/95 mmHg = 0.3) indicating severe flow limitation. Although FFR does not measure coronary flow directly, assumptions can be made in the presence of a hemodynamically significant obstruction. Therefore, adenosine may not cause a large increase in flow in this case, since the lesion is severe at rest. Note there is a minimal change in distal pressure during adenosine-induced hyperemia (the lesion is severely stenotic).

In cases where the resting gradient ratio is not diagnostic, the hyperemic pressure ratio (FFR) should always be calculated.

8. **c** The distal FFR gradually normalizes with pullback of the pressure wire to the segment just distal to the stented region (FFR$_{distal}$ = 0.41, FFR$_{mid}$ = 0.95). This indicates that pressure (and therefore flow) across the stented segment is normalized. Combined with the angiographic images showing diffuse and irregular disease, continuous pullback of the pressure wire reveals a gradual pressure loss across the length of the mid- to distal artery. Distal pressure is often lower than proximal pressure when diffuse disease is present. An abrupt loss of pressure would suggest a focal stenosis accounting for the differences in FFR. Guide catheter damping is not evident based on waveform analysis of the aortic pressure tracings during pullback.

9. **d** The hemodynamic tracing reveals a translesional resting peak–peak pressure gradient of over 120 mmHg, which indicates significant obstruction to flow. However, there are two possible reasons for flow limitation: fixed obstruction or vasospasm. Suspicion for other potential etiologic explanations based on the clinical presentation should prompt the operator to give nitroglycerin and re measure.

10. **b** In this case, significant vasospasm may have occurred during pressure wire passage of the diseased segments. There was no thrombus reported on the initial angiogram and hemodynamic resolution after nitroglycerin injection makes thrombus less likely. Truly obstructive atherosclerotic lesions usually show a significant translesional pressure gradient that persists even after vasodilator (nitroglycerin or adenosine) injection.

The mechanisms for coronary vasospasm are not well understood. Prinzmetal first described variant angina as an unusual form of coronary ischemia, which was not provoked by typical exercise-related factors, and is accompanied by ST-segment elevation. It is known that atherosclerosis interferes with the normal endothelial function and the modulation of resting coronary tone. *In vivo* studies have demonstrated that while acetylcholine dilates the normal coronary artery segment, it produces vasoconstriction in diseased coronary artery segments.

11. **d** Coronary vasospasm is associated with symptoms both at rest and during exertion, often with a circadian pattern. Symptoms commonly occur in the morning hours and abate spontaneously within minutes. They may be prolonged, and if sustained, could be associated with myocardial infarction, high grade AV-block or ventricular arrhythmias.

Sublingual nitroglycerin is effective in aborting the acute episode. High grade AV-block or ventricular arrhythmias are not common during severe vasospasm episodes. If ventricular arrhythmias recur despite medical treatment with calcium channel blocking or nitrate agents, an ICD may be required.

Angina associated with ST-segment depression during stress testing is not an indication for provocative testing with ergonovine. In this setting, obstructive (fixed) coronary artery disease is most likely. The common indications for ergonovine provocation during coronary angiography include strong clinical suspicion of vasospasm with or without ECG changes. In a patient without obstructive coronary artery disease, pain accompanied by ST-elevation at rest with ST-elevation relieved after the event, is considered to be spasm until proven otherwise and does not need ergonovine testing. Ergonovine maleate is an ergot alkaloid that stimulates both α-adrenergic and serotonergic receptors, thereby exerting a direct vasoconstrictive effect on vascular smooth muscle. Coronary arteries that constrict spontaneously appear to be abnormally sensitive to this agent. In low doses and in carefully controlled clinical situations, ergonovine is a relatively safe drug, but prolonged coronary artery vasospasm precipitated by ergonovine has been reported to cause myocardial infarction. Because of this hazard, it is recommended that ergonovine only be administered to patients in whom coronary angiography has documented normal (or nearly normal) coronary arteries—and even then, beginning with a very low dose. Many invasive cardiologists have abandoned ergonovine provocation, opting for empiric medical management with calcium channel blockers when coronary vasospasm is suspected. Ergonovine is FDA approved only for post-partum or post-abortal uterine bleeding, by strengthening the force, duration and frequency of uterine contractions. Although ergonovine is not FDA approved for intracoronary administration, it remains the most commonly used agent for excluding coronary vasospasm.

12. e Transient ST-segment elevation during exercise stress testing is associated occasionally with inducible coronary vasospasm that may be revealed angiographically during ergonovine provocation testing. Resting pain with ST-elevation that improves with pain resolution is diagnostic and does not require further testing. Amenorrhea in pre-menopausal females, severe hypertension, severe LV dysfunction and severe aortic stenosis are all contraindications for ergonovine provocation. In the setting of amenorrhea or dysmenorrhea, acetylcholine can be safely substituted.

13. d Ergonovine induced coronary vasospasm is also common in atherosclerotic coronary arteries, although it produces diffuse narrowing in normal coronary arteries. The sensitivity of the ergonovine provocation increases for recorded ST-segment elevation during rest angina—up to 58% of patients will show a vasospastic response. Inducible vasospasm is observed in only 15% of patients who present with isolated atypical chest pain.

14. d Calcium channel blocking agents have been shown to reduce the incidence of spontaneous and exercise-induced coronary vasospasm and associated ischemic sequelae like ventricular tachycardia (VT). The addition of nitrates may also be effective, if needed. Direct referral for electrophysiologic testing or ICD placement is not appropriate as an initial therapy. β-Blocking agents do not inhibit coronary vasospasm and some older reports indicate β-blockers may exacerbate vasospasm.

Chapter 17

Calculations Used
in Hemodynamics

1. **Which of the following does not adversely affect the measurement of cardiac output (CO) by thermodilution (TD) technique?**
   a. Low CO states
   b. High CO states
   c. The temperature of the injectate saline
   d. Severe tricuspid regurgitation
   e. Severe respiratory variation

2. **The following values were obtained in the catheterization lab. What is the calculated CO?**

Femoral artery O_2 sat = 0.94
Hemoglobin = 14.0 g/dL
Body surface area = 1.8 m²
Pulmonary artery (PA) O_2 sat = 0.73
Oxygen consumption = 240 mL/min

   a. 8.16 L/min
   b. 6.0 L/min
   c. 10.8 L/min
   d. 4.4 L/min
   e. 3.3 L/min

Use the following values obtained in the catheterization lab to answer Questions 3–5.

Femoral artery O_2 sat = 0.94
Hemoglobin = 14.0 g/dL
Body surface area = 1.8 m²
Aortic pressure = 140/75, mean 100 mmHg
Right atrial mean pressure = 10 mmHg
Pulmonary artery O_2 sat = 0.73
Oxygen consumption = 240 mL/min
Cardiac output = 6.0 L/min
PA pressure = 35/15, mean 25 mmHg
PCW mean pressure = 16 mmHg

3. **What is the calculated systemic vascular resistance (SVR)?**
   a. 1200 dyne/s/cm⁻⁵
   b. 1120 dyne/s/cm⁻⁵
   c. 1000 dyne/s/cm⁻⁵
   d. 14.0 Wood units
   e. 12.5 Wood units

4. **What is the total peripheral resistance (TPR)?**
   a. 1466 dyne/s/cm^{-5}
   b. 1333 dyne/s/cm^{-5}
   c. 1200 dyne/s/cm^{-5}
   d. 1120 dyne/s/cm^{-5}
   e. 1000 dyne/s/cm^{-5}

5. **What is the calculated pulmonary vascular resistance (PVR)?**
   a. 12.5 Wood units
   b. 2.5 Wood units
   c. 1.5 Wood units
   d. 200 dyne/s/cm^{-5}
   e. 160 dyne/s/cm^{-3}

A 64-year-old man with severe dyspnea on exertion is referred for cardiac catheterization. Simultaneous left ventricular (LV) and left atrial (LA) tracings are shown on Figure 17.1.

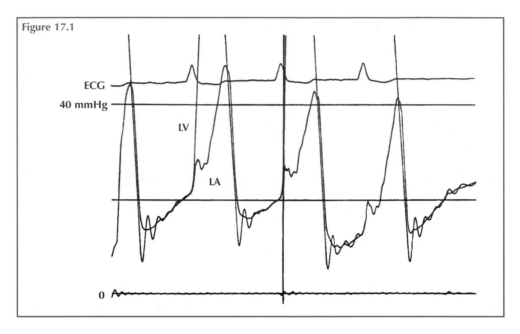

Figure 17.1

The following data are obtained.

Cardiac output (Fick) = 4.6 L/min
End-diastolic LV volume = 175 mL
End-systolic LV volume = 45 mL
Heart rate = 60 bpm
Blood pressure = 110/50
Hemoglobin = 13 g/dL

6. **What is the total stroke volume in this patient?**
   a. 220 mL
   b. 175 mL
   c. 130 mL
   d. 115 mL
   e. 77 mL

7. **What is the ejection fraction?**
   a. 85%
   b. 74%
   c. 66%
   d. 44%
   e. 26%

8. What is the volume of blood ejected into the aorta with each beat (effective stroke volume)?
    a. 175 mL
    b. 130 mL
    c. 115 mL
    d. 77 mL
    e. 38 mL

9. What is the regurgitant volume?
    a. 98 mL
    b. 92 mL
    c. 53 mL
    d. 38 mL
    e. 19 mL

10. What is the regurgitant fraction?
    a. 74%
    b. 53%
    c. 49%
    d. 41%
    e. 29%

11. Based on your calculations, this patient's mitral regurgitation is classified as:
    a. Mild
    b. Moderate
    c. Moderate to severe
    d. Severe
    e. Critical

Answers

1. **b** CO, when measured by TD techniques, is affected by conditions that limit the flow of the injectate saline from the proximal port on the catheter to the temperature probe. Severe tricuspid regurgitation makes the measurement unreliable. Low CO states may cause a change in the injectate temperature due to warming by the walls of the cardiac chambers. Respiratory variation may cause changes in baseline temperature of blood in the pulmonary artery. The magnitude of this intrinsic temperature change can approach the change measured as a result of the cold indicator injection. The effect of the injectate saline temperature is negligible, provided that the correct computational constants are used for the calculations. The manufacturer provides the computational constants for each device, which vary with both the temperature and the volume of the injectate saline bolus.

2. **b** CO = $[(O_2$ consumption) / $(FAO_2 - PAO_2)] \times Hb \times (O_2$ capacity/g Hb) $\times 10$
   = $[240$ mL/min / $(0.94 - 0.73)] \times (14$ g/dL$) \times (1.36$ mL O_2/g Hb$) \times 10$
   = 6.0 L/min
   Cardiac index = CO / body surface area
   = 6.0 L/min/1.8m^2
   = 3.3 L/min/m^2

   Extraction of nutrients by metabolizing tissues is a function of the rate of blood delivery and the rate of tissue extraction from the circulation. Tissue viability can be maintained despite a fall in CO as long as there is an increased extraction capability for required nutrients. Delivery of blood to tissue is grossly measured as CO. The range of normal CO is influenced by several variables, the most important of which is body size. Oxygen consumption and metabolic rate correlate best with body surface area (BSA). Thus, CO is often normalized to BSA. Net forward flow (i.e. CO) is then reported as CO/BSA, or cardiac index. Although the body's metabolic rate declines with increasing age, no further correction for age is necessary. Other factors affecting CO include posture, body temperature, anxiety, environmental heat and humidity.

   Of the many techniques devised to determine CO, only two are generally accepted in clinical practice: the Fick oxygen technique and the indicator-dilution technique. In the Fick method, pulmonary blood flow (which is equal to systemic blood flow in the absence of shunts) is determined by measuring the arteriovenous oxygen difference across the lungs and the rate of oxygen uptake by blood from the lungs (i.e. oxygen consumption). Thus, CO = oxygen consumption/arteriovenous oxygen difference. In most laboratories, oxygen consumption is measured using a metabolic cart.

   There are two general types of indicator-dilution methods: the continuous-infusion method and the single-injection method. Both methods require the injectate to mix completely with the blood, and that the injectate is neither added nor subtracted from the blood between injection and sampling sites. Historically, indocyanine green dye was injected into the pulmonary artery and then detected in a peripheral system artery. This material has been replaced with the TD method, in which the injectate is a 'cold' saline bolus that is injected into the right atrium. The re-warmed blood (i.e. temperature change) is sensed in the pulmonary artery. Rare but severe allergic reactions have been described with indocyanine green dye, mostly in patients with renal failure. Indocyanine green dye is no longer manufactured for clinical use.

The TD technique is susceptible to several pitfalls. Because the data represent right-sided CO, tricuspid regurgitation can be a problem as the saline bolus is interrupted. The TD method tends to overestimate CO in low-output states, because the dissipation of the cooler temperature to the surrounding cardiac structures results in a reduced measured temperature, resulting in a falsely elevated CO. Other sources of error include respiratory fluctuations in blood temperature and the gradual warming of the saline injectate prior to actual injection. Computational constants allow for the use of either ice-bath immersion or room-temperature saline boluses. Because variability between measurements can be relatively large, at least three determinations should be averaged, and small changes should not be over-interpreted. CO data from the TD technique are accurate only to within a 15% error.

CO can also be estimated from angiography using the equation:

(ventricular stroke volume/beat) x heart rate

Although angiographic stroke volume can be calculated by tracing the end-diastolic and end-systolic images following ventriculography, the inherent inaccuracies of calibrating angiographic volumes often make this measurement method difficult, if not unreliable. In cases of valvular regurgitation or atrial fibrillation, angiographic CO will not accurately reflect true CO.

3. a Systemic vascular resistance (SVR) in absolute units is calculated using the equation:

SVR $= [80 \times (\text{Ao mean} - \text{RA mean})] / Qs$, where Qs = systemic flow in L/min
SVR $= [80 \times (100 - 10)] / 6 = 1200$ dyne/s/cm^5

The constant (80) is used to convert units from mmHg/L/min (Wood units) to the absolute resistance unit dyne/s/cm^5.

To convert SVR to SVRI:

SVRI $=$ SVR / BSA (m^2)
$= 1200/1.8$ m$^2 = 666$ dyne/s/cm^5/m^2

Vascular resistance calculations are based on hydraulic principles of fluid flow, in which resistance is defined as the ratio of the decrease in pressure between two points in a vascular segment and the blood flow through that segment. Although analogous to Ohm's law, this represents an over-simplification of the complex behavior of pulsatile flow in dynamic vascular beds. Nonetheless, the calculated vascular resistance has proven to be of value in a number of clinical settings. Elevated resistances in the systemic and pulmonary circuits may represent reversible abnormalities or may be fixed due to irreversible anatomic changes.

Vascular impedance measurements account for blood viscosity, pulsatile flow, reflected waves and arterial compliance. These measurements have the potential to accurately describe the dynamic pressure-flow relationship more comprehensively than using simplistic vascular resistance calculations. However, impedance data are complex and difficult to obtain, and as a result, impedance measurement has not been adopted as a routine clinical practice in most laboratories.

4. b If the right atrial mean pressure is not known, its value can be dropped from the equation as shown:

$$TPR = [80 \times Ao\ mean] / Qs$$
$$= [80 \times 100] / 6 = 1333\ dyne/s/cm^{-5}$$

5. c Similarly, pulmonary vascular resistance is derived using the mean PA and mean LA pressures:

$$PVR = [80\ (PA\ mean - LA\ mean)] / Qp,\ where\ Qp = pulmonary\ flow\ in\ L/min$$
$$= [80\ (25 - 16)] / 6 = 120\ dyne/s/cm^{-5},\ or\ 1.5\ Wood\ units$$

In the absence of an intracardiac shunt, Qp is equal to Qs.

6. c Total stroke volume (SV) = end-diastolic volume (EDV) - end-systolic volume (ESV)
$$= 175\ mL - 45\ mL$$
$$= 130\ mL$$

This is sometimes referred to as the angiographic stroke volume. With the degree of mitral regurgitation present, it is incorrect to calculate stroke volume by dividing CO by the heart rate.

7. b Ejection fraction
$$= (EDV - ESV) / EDV$$
$$= SV / EDV$$
$$= 130\ mL / 175\ mL$$
$$= 0.74\ or\ 74\%$$

8. d Effective stroke volume
$$= CO / heart\ rate$$
$$= (4600\ mL/min) / 60\ beats/min$$
$$= 77\ mL$$

This is sometimes referred to as the forward stroke volume.

The information needed to calculate regurgitant volume and regurgitant fraction is readily available in the catheterization laboratory. The most common method for angiographically calculating ventricular volumes is to assume that the ventricle is an ellipsoid, using dimensions from biplane left ventriculography. A correction must be made for the degree of magnification incurred during the imaging process, using an object of known size (such as a standardized grid or phantom) at the level of the heart, and then applying a correction factor (which must be cubed when calculating a volume).

Once the angiographic end-diastolic and end-systolic volumes are calculated, the angiographic (or total) stroke volume can be calculated (and multiplied by the heart rate to determine the angiographic CO). Forward stroke volume is calculated by dividing the forward CO (determined by TD or the Fick method) by the heart rate. The difference between the angiographic stroke volume and the forward stroke volume is the regurgitant stroke volume. The regurgitant fraction is then easily calculated by dividing the regurgitant volume by the angiographic stroke volume.

9. c Regurgitant volume = total stroke volume - effective stroke volume
$$= 130 \text{ mL} - 77 \text{ mL}$$
$$= 53 \text{ mL}$$

In patients with aortic and/or mitral regurgitation, a comparison between angiographic stroke volume and forward stroke volume (or effective stroke volume) provides an estimation of the volume (and severity) of the ejected volume that is regurgitated, and thus does not contribute to the net CO. Because the calculated regurgitant volume or fraction requires the comparison of two different methods for stroke volume measurement, both of which contain some degree of error, the net overall degree of error is magnified. Interpretation of either regurgitant volume or regurgitant fraction should be influenced by another qualitative assessment, such as echocardiography or cineangiography. This is particularly true in cases of combined aortic and mitral regurgitation.

10. d Regurgitant fraction = regurgitant volume / total stroke volume
$$= 53 \text{ mL} / 130 \text{ mL}$$
$$= 0.41 \text{ or } 41\%$$

11. c A regurgitant fraction of 40–60% is considered moderate to severe.

Regurgitant fraction	Severity of regurgitation
<20%	Mild
20–40%	Moderate
40–60%	Moderate to severe
>60%	Severe

2-D	2-dimensional
Ao	aortic
AoR	aortic root
AR	aortic regurgitation
AS	aortic stenosis
ASD	atrial septal defect
AV	atrioventricular
AVA	aortic valve area
BP	blood pressure
BSA	body surface area
CAD	coronary artery disease
CHF	congestive heart failure
CI	cardiac index
CO	cardiac output
COPD	chronic obstructive pulmonary disease
CVR	coronary flow velocity reserve
ECG	electrocardiogram
EDV	end-diastolic volume
ESV	end-systolic volume
FA	femoral artery
FFR	fractional flow reserve
HCM	hypertrophic cardiomyopathy
HR	heart rate
IABP	intra-aortic balloon pump
ICD	intracoronary device
ICU	intensive care unit
IVRT	isovolumic relaxation time
IVUS	intravascular ultrasound
LA	left atrium/left atrial
LAD	left anterior descending
LMCA	left main coronary artery
LV	left ventricle/left ventricular
LVEDP	left ventricular end-diastolic pressure
LVEF	left ventricular ejection fraction
LVOT	left ventricular outflow tract
MR	mitral regurgitation
MS	mitral stenosis
MVO_2	mixed venous oxygen content
NPV	negative predictive value
NTG	nitroglycerin
NYHA	New York Heart Association
PA	pulmonary artery
PAC	premature atrial contraction
PAP	pulmonary artery pressure
PASP	pulmonary artery systolic pressure
PBV	pulmonary balloon valvuloplasty
PCW	pulmonary capillary wedge
PDA	posterior descending artery
PFO	patent foramen ovale
PPV	positive predictive value

PRU	peripheral resistance units
PS	pulmonary stenosis
PSVT	paroxysmal supraventricular tachycardia
PTCA	percutaneous transluminal coronary angioplasty
PTSMA	percutaneous transluminal septal myocardial ablation
PVC	premature ventricular contraction
PVR	pulmonary vascular resistance
PVRI	pulmonary vascular resistance index
Qp	pulmonary blood flow
Qs	systemic blood flow
RA	right atrium/right atrial
RAP	right atrial pressure
RCA	right coronary artery
RCVR	relative coronary flow velocity reserve
RF	regurgitant fraction
RHD	rheumatic heart disease
RV	right ventricle/right ventricular
RVEDP	right ventricular end-diastolic pressure
RVOT	right ventricular outflow tract
RVSP	right ventricular systolic pressure
SA	systemic arterial
SEP	systolic ejection period
SV	stroke volume
SVR	systemic vascular resistance
TD	thermodilution
TPR	total peripheral resistance
TR	tricuspid regurgitation
TS	tricuspid stenosis
TV	tricuspid valve
VSD	ventricular septal defect
VT	ventricular tachycardia